THE KNEE CRISIS HANDBOOK

"Dr. Halpern masterfully describes the essence of good knee health. He clearly — and most importantly, accurately — explains how to recognize when the knee is not healthy, and then how to get it healthy and keep it healthy. As a leading sports medicine physician and former president of the American Medical Society of Sports Medicine, Dr. Halpern's passion towards his work, and his compassionate and humorous bedside manner, resonate clearly."

CINDY J. CHANG, M.D.
HEAD TEAM PHYSICIAN, UNIVERSITY OF CALIFORNIA AT BERKELEY

"While there have been many other books written about the knee, few have been written about the patient with knee problems. *The Knee Crisis Handbook* provides valuable guidelines and insight into constructing diagnosis and treatment strategies; it gives the patient the power to find a doctor, understand diagnostic tests and manage treatment. Dr. Halpern's approach is based on the family practice model of addressing a problem in the context of the total person."

STANLEY A. HERRING, M.D.
TEAM PHYSICIAN, SEATTLE SEAHAWKS
CLINICAL PROFESSOR, DEPARTMENT OF REHABILITATION MEDICINE/
DEPARTMENT OF ORTHOPEDICS, UNIVERSITY OF WASHINGTON

"This book is all about plain talk and advice. This is what your physician should be telling you, but either doesn't have the time or the inclination to do so. This is not a book of conjecture, just plain practical tips based upon scientific evidence. There are a lot of physicians who could learn a great deal from this volume. I would point out the superb chapter on the Sport-by-Sport Health Guide. It was wonderfully done. My congratulations to Dr. Halpern."

DOUGLAS B. MCKEAG, M.D., M.S.
AUL PROFESSOR OF PREVENTATIVE HEALTH MEDICINE
CHAIR, DEPARTMENT OF FAMILY MEDICINE
DIRECTOR, INDIANA UNIVERSITY CENTER FOR SPORTS MEDICINE

"Dr. Halpern draws on his many years of experience with patients – from couch potatoes to elite athletes – in this easy-to-follow, comprehensive guide to knee pain. It's a "must read" for anyone considering knee surgery!"

LISA R. CALLAHAN, M.D.
AUTHOR, THE FITNESS FACTOR

"*The Knee Crisis Handbook* is a comprehensive and authoritative guide for knee care. Dr. Halpern has authored the state-of-the-art text for understanding everything about the knee. From prevention of injuries, to understanding how to make the diagnosis, to treatment of specific problems, this text has a wealth of information. It just might save you a visit to the emergency room."

E. LEE RICE, D.O.
SAN DIEGO SPORTS MEDICINE

"*The Knee Crisis Handbook* is an excellent resource that patients can use to guide them through the complexities of a knee injury. It is clearly written, concise and up-to-date. I think that patients will find it useful in helping them partner with their physician as they work together to heal their injury."

JAMES C. PUFFER, M.D.
FORMER HEAD PHYSICIAN OF THE 1988 UNITED STATES SUMMER OLYMPIC TEAM AND
PHYSICIAN TO THE 1984 UNITED STATES WINTER OLYMPIC TEAM

Dr. Brian Halpern has translated a very complicated and important part of the musculoskeletal system to terms that can be understood by anyone. His conversational style gives the reader the feeling of being in his office discussing the problems. This practical presentation of the knee would be a beneficial reference to any home with physically active individuals.

JOHN A. LOMBARDO, M.D.
PROFESSOR, DEPARTMENT OF FAMILY MEDICINE, OHIO STATE UNIVERSITY
MEDICAL DIRECTOR OF OHIO STATE UNIVERSITY SPORTS MEDICINE CENTER
HEAD TEAM PHYSICIAN, OSU ATHLETIC DEPARTMENT

THE KNEE CRISIS HANDBOOK

Understanding Pain, Preventing Trauma,
Recovering from Injury, and
Building Healthy Knees for Life

BY BRIAN HALPERN, M.D.
WITH LAURA TUCKER

FOREWORD BY JACK C. HUGHSTON, M.D.
INTRODUCTION BY JANE E. BRODY

RODALE

The Knee Crisis Handbook: Understanding Pain, Preventing Trauma, Recovering from Injury, and Building Healthy Knees for Life

Internet addresses and telephone numbers given in this book were accurate at the time it went to press.

© 2003 LifeTime Media, Inc.
A LifeTime Media Production
LifeTime Media, Inc.
352 Seventh Avenue, 15th Floor
New York, NY 10001

Illustrations © 2003 LifeTime Media, Inc.
Knee Aspiration cartoon © 2003, Hughston Sports Medicine Foundation, Inc. Reprinted with permission from the publisher.
All X-Rays and MRIs © 1997, Blackwell Publishing. Reprinted with permission from the publisher.

Printed in the United States of America

Rodale Inc. makes every effort to use acid-free ∞, recycled paper ♲ .

Illustrations by Laura Siegel
Book design by Amy V. Wilson

Library of Congress Cataloging-in-Publication Data

Halpern, Brian.
    The knee crisis handbook : understanding pain, preventing trauma, recovering from injury, and building healthy knees for life / Brian Halpern, with Laura Tucker ; foreword by Jack C. Hughston ; introduction by Jane E. Brody.
        p.   cm.
    Includes bibliographical references and index.
    ISBN 1–57954–871–7 paperback
    1. Knee—Care and hygiene.   2. Knee—Wounds and injuries—Prevention.
I. Tucker, Laura. II. Title.
RD561.H355   2004
617.5'82—dc22   2003018371

Distributed to the book trade by St. Martin's Press

  4 6 8 10 9 7 5 3   paperback

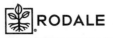

RODALE

WE **INSPIRE** AND **ENABLE** PEOPLE TO IMPROVE
THEIR LIVES AND THE WORLD AROUND THEM

FOR MORE OF OUR PRODUCTS
WWW.RODALESTORE.COM
(800) 848-4735

DEDICATION

Dedicated to the memory of Stephen Hunter, M.D., visionary, caring physician, mentor, and friend.

To my wife, Karen, and daughters, Danyelle, Samantha, and Alyson, and my parents, Dwight and Rosalie Halpern. Thanks for all of your patience and help.

To my office staff in New York and New Jersey, thanks for always being there.

To my patients who volunteered their time and stories and have helped me to be a better doctor, thank you.

ACKNOWLEDGMENTS

For their expert advice and support, thank you to David Altchek, M.D., Sports Orthopedic Surgeon, and Sergio Schwartzman, M.D., Rheumatologist. Thanks also to LifeTime Media, Jeremy Katz at Rodale, and my co-author, Laura Tucker. Thanks especially to Marty Jaramillo, P.T., A.T.C., C.S.C.S., and Robert Abramson, M.D., for their contributions to the book.

CONTENTS

FOREWORD

The Knee Crisis Handbook is an excellent book, presented to benefit the reader, whether a layperson or a professional. It is valuable to anyone involved in athletic training, coaching, physical fitness, physical therapy, or medicine—either as a patient or a practitioner.

The section on "Preventing Knee Injury" reflects much of the progress that has been made in this area over the last twenty years, especially the importance of proper training. The "Psychological Effects of Knee Injury" uses a commonsense approach to address a subject not often covered. Most important, this book treats the body as a whole, stressing the critical relationship of overall health and fitness to the health and fitness of the knee.

I am going to take some secondhand credit for the quality you see here. Brian Halpern was the first family physician to perform the Fellowship in Sports Medicine, the brainchild of Dr. Stephen Hunter of our Hughston Sports Medicine Foundation. Dr. Hunter's program has gained considerable importance in the field and has been duplicated in many orthopedic/sports medicine training centers. Dr. Brian Halpern was the first, and he has represented and expanded the field of Sports Medicine nobly.

This book is accessible and most informative, clearly the result of the author's vast experience. My congratulations to Brian Halpern on this book.

Jack C. Hughston, M.D.

INTRODUCTION

By Jane E. Brody

Personal Health Columnist, The New York Times

only wish I'd had this book thirty-five years ago – before I became a runner, a fanatical tennis player, a downhill skier. Before I'd torn three ligaments, tore and shredded a meniscus, and developed advanced arthritis in both knees because I didn't know enough about strength training and stretching.

If I'd been able to read and apply the simple and sensible advice in this book, I would have known how to protect these most valuable joints in my body so that now, in my sixties, I'd still be able to hold my own on the tennis court, zip around the skating rink, walk painlessly down a flight of stairs and just walk—as long and as far as I may want to.

I wish I'd known thirty-five years ago just how often I put myself at increased risk of knee injury, and that the wear-and-tear arthritis that now cramps my lifestyle will eventually mean a double knee replacement.

The Knee Crisis Handbook by Dr. Brian Halpern is loaded with invaluable information on protecting and rehabilitating knees, information that is accessible to any reader interested in pursuing health and remaining physically active from cradle to grave. It is filled with facts and practical advice from a real pro that you're not likely to find anywhere else, certainly not all in one place.

The book is extremely helpful to those who, like me, have already sustained serious knee damage and now face the prospect of rehabilitation, surgery, or both. You will learn how to postpone the day when you may be forced by disability to undergo surgery, and what to do if and when that day should come. You will learn why you should not ignore knee pain until it becomes crippling.

You will also learn something else I wish I'd known years ago—how to choose and evaluate a physical therapist who really knows knees and knows how to get an injured or surgical patient back on track and moving again in a way that protects against reinjury. A good therapist should be able to motivate you to continue on your own to do the work necessary to keep your knees healthy.

The knee is a joint that evolution never finished improving. If you could look through the files of any orthopedic surgeon, it would be immediately apparent that the human knee was simply not designed to withstand the stresses of modern life. Once primates started walking on two instead of four legs, two instead of four knees were forced to bear the body's full weight and adjust to every twist and turn, jump and squat, along with such routine stresses as climbing up and down stairs and bending over to pick up something on the floor.

Just think how many times a day you flex, rotate, pivot, extend, shift, lean, walk, run, jump, kneel, or otherwise use and abuse your knees. And that is not to mention the abuse sustained through years of dancing, jogging, skiing, gardening, cycling, golfing, playing tennis, in-line skating, spring cleaning, even swimming. Almost everything people do for recreation is tough on the knee.

From one perspective, the knee is a remarkable feat of engineering, a highly complex joint with an incredible range of motion. But it is also a rather small joint, considering the burden it must bear and the tasks it is asked daily to perform. This renders the knee highly vulnerable to injury. It is a joint that was designed to last maybe forty years, not the eighty or more most of us now are living.

You don't have to be skiing moguls or playing Ultimate Frisbee to sustain a serious knee injury. Simply missing a step or doing too many whip kicks in the pool can do it. This makes it important for everyone to know how to strengthen the muscles that support the knee to reduce its burden.

The Knee Crisis Handbook will tell you exactly how—and why—this should be done. It explains, for example, why a cyclist with highly developed thigh muscles may still be at risk of a knee injury because his muscle development is unbalanced. It will convince you of the critical necessity of regular stretching exercises to reduce the risk that overly tight muscles will cause a tear in a ligament or tendon stressed beyond its limits.

Everyone who is physically active—and everyone who is inactive— should read this book. So that means everyone, since both the active and inactive are at risk of suffering debilitating knee injuries that can keep them from enjoying the best things in life—from a walk in the country to carrying a grandchild. How do you explain to a tired eighteen-month-old that you cannot carry him up the stairs because your knees hurt?

So please don't wait until you yourself are suffering a "knee crisis" before you read this book and apply the lessons herein. You'll be very glad you did.

PART I

THE KNEE

THE KNEE CRISIS

There is a knee crisis in America. People are experiencing more injuries—and more serious injuries—to their knees than ever before. The frequency of knee pain and knee joint replacements has skyrocketed, including those in Americans under the age of sixty. As a culture, we're putting a tremendous strain on one of our most important joints, with potentially debilitating results.

There are many reasons for the increase in knee pain. Knee traumas in women, especially, have gone up dramatically, and recent statistical analysis shows that women are four to six times more likely to have specific traumatic knee injuries (like ligament tears) than men are. As more and more women experience the joy and health benefits of an active lifestyle and competitive sports, the incidence of injury is only going to increase.

Sports like soccer and basketball are rising in popularity, especially in recreational leagues. These also happen to be two of the sports with the highest rate of knee incident. Weekend warriors are pushing their bodies harder and further, past what they can safely do. This is especially true of middle-aged exercisers who, after years of physical activity, have put many miles on their knees on the bike, the road, or the trail. Many of these athletes choose to ignore the first signs of problems and "play through the pain." This puts them at higher risk for serious injury, as well as degeneration later in life.

Conversely, we're more out of shape than we've ever been in this country. A large segment of the population is sedentary and under-conditioned. For every "overuse" injury I treat, I see as many problems that are the result of "underuse," in someone so poorly conditioned and overweight that even the normal activities of daily living put an undue strain on the knees. It's not just biking a hundred miles that can wear down the knees; in the wrong circumstances, just walking to the car (or not walking to the car enough) can bring on knee pain.

We're also seeing an increase in degenerative knee pain and injury. At least some of this is linked to previous knee injury, whether from trauma or overuse, that puts you at higher risk for degenerative conditions such as arthritis. This is also linked to what has been called "the graying of America"—as the population gets older and lives longer, our bodies have more time to wear down and wear out.

The knee injury rate is on the rise in this country and surgery is keeping pace. Making a decision about surgery should be a complicated decision, and one made on a patient-by-patient basis, as both the patient and the physician weigh the particulars of the specific knee problem and the individual's long-term health and goals.

Cutting-edge imaging techniques give us fantastic access to the inner anatomy of the knee and can be an invaluable aid when we are trying to locate the source of your pain, and surgery has had life-changing effects on many of my patients. Surgeries have become much easier to perform, with fewer complications and inconveniences. Procedures that used to take hours and require months of immobilization can now be performed on an outpatient basis, so that the patient is up and around in a matter of days.

However, these amazing technologies cannot and should not be treated as a substitute for good old-fashioned, hands-on doctoring. These imaging techniques should be used to *supplement* the information we get from an examination, not *supplant* it, and surgical options should be used to complement intelligent, active participation in your personal knee health, not as a substitute for it.

I know, both from firsthand experience and from seeing thousands of patients over the course of my career, that any pain or injury in the knee is a crisis for the person who's experiencing it. A sore or injured knee directly interferes with our ability to live our lives the way we want to, because the knee is the basis for our mobility. An injured knee can mean you can't enjoy that skiing vacation, or achieve your life-long goal of reaching the top of Kilimanjaro. When your knee hurts, you can't run to catch a bus, or climb a ladder, or squat to comfort a child. You can't even sit comfortably in front of a computer to do your job— or drive a stick-shift car to get there.

Even if it's only slight discomfort, knee pain is a serious matter that should be addressed. A knee injury affects our ability to bend and straighten our leg, something everyone does thousands of times every day, but the consequences extend far past the joint. A knee injury can put the rest of the body in danger by forcing you to compensate for your weakness. And it makes it harder to do the exercise that keeps our hearts and lungs and bodies healthy and strong. Knee injuries aren't cheap, either—from what you spend on braces and orthotics and physical therapy, to the money you lose on a business deal because you're stuck in the clubhouse with an icepack instead of out on the links.

And then there's an emotional and psychological cost. We understand our ability to move under our own steam and without pain as a fundamental entitlement. Any restriction placed on that ability affects our confidence and our general state of mind. If you're someone who jogs to clear your head after a tough day, catches up with friends over a pickup game of basketball, or spends the weekend Rollerblading with your kids, a knee injury can drastically interfere with your sense of mental well-being.

In the case of a traumatic knee injury, getting the right diagnosis and care is absolutely essential in making a full recovery, and in this book, I will equip you with the information you need to make educated decisions about your care. In many cases, the advent of a serious knee problem is slow in coming, with many signs along the way, and there is much that can be done to strengthen the structures that support this essential joint. One of the keys to knee health, then, is to listen to your body and understand the signs of impending trouble. I can help you do that—and help you to know when you should take action.

Doctors may have told you that if your chosen activity causes you pain, then you should give it up. This doesn't have to be true. Your hobbies are an important part of what makes your life enjoyable, and the health benefits of an active lifestyle need to be weighed against the cost to your knee. In some cases, I may advise you to take a break, and I may advise you to modify your activity to address your personal anatomical or physical limitations. In general, however, I believe that the key to knee health is to exercise in a *proper and intelligent manner*. I want you to be jogging, hiking, or playing tennis twenty years from now without any pain at all.

I am writing this book because I know that, one patient at a time, we can put a stop to the knee crisis in this country. The secret is to start treating the underlying problem, not just the symptoms—the whole patient, not just the joint. In order to make this happen, I want to empower you to take control of your knee health.

What are the factors putting you at risk for knee injury, and what can you do to offset some of those risks? What sport-specific measures should you be taking to make sure that you're playing as safely as possible? When and how should you seek medical attention for knee pain and discomfort? How will you know you're being guided to the best treatment for your particular injury, or given the right alternatives to surgery? If surgery is the best option, what should you expect—before, during, and after the procedure? What should you look for in a physical therapist, and what exercises can you do on your own to strengthen an injured knee? And, most important, how can you stay as healthy, strong, and pain-free as long as possible?

The body has tremendous healing potential. When you take an active role in your knee health, in cooperation with a doctor who understands your personal history and needs, you are taking an important step toward enjoying the rest of your life to the fullest extent possible.

CHAPTER TWO

HELP! IT HURTS!

K nee pain is uncomfortable, and injuries flat-out hurt. But don't dismiss that pain as a mere annoyance. It's actually a very important clue as to the nature of your injury, your body's way of telling you what's wrong.

Without pain, you'd continue to use your knee until it was completely broken. So pain isn't just nature's sadism at work, it's a form of communication—your body sending up an alert flare. Use the Quick Pain Self-Assessment tool below to determine whether or not you should make a doctor's appointment, go directly to the emergency room, or try some first-aid remedies and preventive measures for a few days to see if your symptoms subside on their own. No matter what you decide, I'll give you the tools you need to manage the pain you feel in the meantime.

Whether your knee pain came on gradually or was the result of a trauma, you may not need to see the doctor just yet; you may be able to get by with the information contained in this chapter. If your pain continues unabated or gets worse after two to three days on the therapy described, or if the pain becomes intolerable at any point, call your doctor. Here are guidelines for accessing your pain:

QUICK PAIN SELF-ASSESSMENT

 DOES THE PAIN FEEL MORE LIKE A TOOTHACHE THAN A STAB? If the answer is yes, read this chapter.

 HAVE YOU EXPERIENCED THIS PAIN BEFORE IN THE SAME SITE, AND DID IT GO AWAY WITHOUT TREATMENT? If the answer is yes, read this chapter.

 IS THE PAIN CONSTANT OR INTERMITTENT? If the pain is intermittent, read this chapter. If it's constant, or if the periods of intermittent pain are debilitating and come often, call your doctor.

 CAN YOU BEAR WEIGHT ON THE LIMB? If the answer is yes, read this chapter. If the answer is no, call your doctor immediately and describe your symptoms.

 DOES THE KNEE APPEAR TO BE IMPROVING? If it feels better than it did yesterday, read this chapter. If the answer is no—it's worse, or hasn't improved over a day or two—call your doctor and describe your symptoms.

 HAVE YOU BEEN RUNNING A FEVER SINCE THE ONSET OF THE PAIN? If yes, call your doctor immediately. This may be a sign of related infection and can be serious if left untreated.

 IS YOUR KNEE GIVING OUT OR BUCKLING? If yes, call your doctor.

 IS THE KNEE BADLY BRUISED OR BLEEDING? If yes, call your doctor.

➲ **DOES THE PAIN WAKE YOU AT NIGHT?** If yes, call your doctor.

➲ **DOES YOUR KNEE LOCK IN PLACE?** If yes, call your doctor.

➲ **IS THE KNEE SWOLLEN SO THAT YOU CAN'T BEND IT OR COMFORTABLY SUPPORT WEIGHT?** If yes, call your doctor.

➲ **DOES THE KNEE APPEAR DEFORMED FROM AN INJURY?** If yes, go to the emergency room.

➲ **HAVE YOU LOST FEELING IN THE FOOT, OR THE LEG BELOW THE INJURED KNEE?** If yes, go to the emergency room.

Coping with Your Pain

Depending on the results of this assessment, you're either on your way to the emergency room, waiting for a doctor's appointment, or have decided to give it a couple of days to heal on its own before you start calling the professionals. But what are you going to do about your discomfort in the meantime?

The standard "prescription" that every physician gives a patient with knee pain is called **RICE**, an acronym that stands for **R**(est), **I**(ce), **C**(ompression), **E**(levation). These work best in combination with one another.

REST

There's an old joke among physicians that goes like this: "Doc, it hurts when I squat." The doctor answers, "Then stop squatting."

Sometimes people have to pay a doctor to tell them what they already know. Here's a freebie: when you're hurt, the first order of business is to relieve the load on the injured joint, and that means eliminating activities that cause pain. If it hurts, don't do it. Depending on the injury, that can mean not jogging for a couple of days, not going up stairs, or not putting any weight on the offending leg at all, by relying on crutches or a cane.

I also want to introduce you to the concept of *relative rest*. You don't want to immobilize the leg for too long—controlled movement promotes healing. But moving too much too fast can make the injury worse. Pain is your body's way of telling you that you need to protect the joint or you'll sustain further injury. Don't ignore the warning signs! Once you've relieved the stress on the joint, preventing further injury and giving your body a little time to rest and recover on its own, we can actually find out what the underlying problem is.

I know it sounds as if I'm contradicting myself when I urge you to stay off the injured knee as well as to move it as soon and as much as you can. The truth is that there's no hard and fast rule for when it's safe or beneficial to move an injured joint: the amount of pain you feel is the best barometer. So you may have to do a little experimenting to see when you're ready, using pain as your guide. Start with the most gentle range-of-motion exercises, like ankle rolls, and slowly straightening and bending your leg. Only go as far as you can without pain—if that's only a matter of a couple of degrees, fine.

Sometimes gentle movement will make an injury feel better. The body "splints" itself when it's injured, immobilizing the painful joint as if it were in a cast. It's a natural tendency: when movement hurts, your body's instinct is to stop the movement. But splinting can really exhaust your muscles, and often when you release their stranglehold on your knee movement, it not only isn't as painful as you'd antici-pated, but it also helps to relieve some of the tension in those muscles.

If movement does hurt, stop moving for a little while and try it again later.

ICE

The use of cold reduces swelling and bleeding, and works as a comfort measure to relieve pain. Reducing swelling promotes healing: a swollen joint is an immobile joint, and an immobile joint is slow to heal.

Reducing swelling also reduces pain. Swelling puts pressure on the pain receptors in the knee. Of course, ice also has a nerve-numbing effect, which can provide you with a nice break from the discomfort you've been feeling!

What should you use to ice your knee? A bag full of ice cubes will work, although a bag of frozen peas is even better. More expensive devices called cryo-cuffs allow you to control the amount of cold on the knee and have compression benefits as well, but they're expensive and unnecessary outside of a locker room or medical facility.

I recommend that you ice the injured leg for 10 to 20 minutes every couple of hours where it's swollen. And I don't hold with the common wisdom that ice is only effective 24 hours after the injury or pain develops. As far as I'm concerned, you can and should ice the joint as long as you have swelling or discomfort from the injury.

> **WARNING:** Icing can actually give you frostbite and tissue damage. Do stop if the skin turns white or bluish, always protect the skin with a towel or cloth, and don't fall asleep while you're icing.

> **A word about heat:** I don't suggest the use of heat for knee injury treatment except in certain specific situations like arthritis pain relief (we'll discuss these situations when we get to them). Heat increases the amount of blood flow into the joint, which can exacerbate swelling, causing more pain.

COMPRESSION

Compression, especially in combination with ice and elevation, can help to prevent or reduce swelling. It may also help to prevent pain by keeping the joint supported and aligned. Short-term immobilization braces or sports wraps can be helpful in keeping the joint still during the rest period immediately after the injury (remember, we want to get the joint moving as soon as possible, so don't get too comfortable in that brace).

The cryo-cuffs I mentioned before combine cold with compression, but you can get the same results at home with a slip-on cuff available from a drugstore (the kind with a hole cut out for the kneecap) and a pack of frozen peas on top. I don't recommend Ace bandages—they're too easy to put on incorrectly.

> **WARNING:** At no point should the compression be painful or cause tingling or throbbing or numbness or swelling in the leg below the bandage or the toes. If this occurs, remove the bandage or sleeve immediately.

ELEVATION

When you're sitting or lying down, it usually helps to elevate the injured knee to the level of or above the heart. This helps to combat swelling, since gravity will ensure that any fluid that might otherwise gather in the knee continues to circulate in your system.

You can use pillows to elevate the leg while you're sitting, sleeping, or watching television.

The components of RICE work best in combination with one another, and with the medications we'll discuss next.

Medications

Whether you're treating pain after an injury or surgery, chronic pain from arthritis, or soreness after a good long hike, a number of medications can help. Some people are more responsive to certain medications than others, so you may need to experiment a little to find the one that works best for your pain.

Questions to Ask Your Doctor Before Taking Medications

Before you take any oral medication, whether over-the-counter or prescription, here are some questions to ask your doctor:

❯ Do I need to take this medication with food or beverage?

❯ Do I need to take it at a specific time of day?

❯ What are the side effects I should look out for?

❯ Will it keep me awake?

❯ Will I experience fewer side effects if I take it before bed?

❯ How does it interact with my other drugs?

❯ Will it make me gain weight?

❯ Can I drink alcohol while I'm on this medication?

You should also give your doctor a full list of all the medications, supplements, vitamins, herbal therapies you take. Some drugs should not be taken with other medications—and remember, just because something's natural or over-the-counter doesn't mean it's harmless in combination with other drugs.

TOPICAL CREAMS

There are any number of topical solutions in the form of creams, liniments, rubs, and sprays available over-the-counter that may help your pain. Some of them use ingredients like camphor or menthol to mask pain via a "counterirritant" effect—the irritation they cause your skin distracts the brain from the pain in the joint. Some creams contain salicylates, the leading ingredient in aspirin, which is something to be mindful of if you're taking aspirin orally (you may want to use the cream and the pills on alternate days). Other creams and liniments include capsaicin, the ingredient that makes chili peppers hot. It heats the skin, and actually blocks a chemical called Substance P, which delivers pain messages to the brain. These creams need to be rubbed into the skin a number of times a day—you may have to use it for a week or more before noticing significant improvement. Wash your hands very carefully before touching your eyes or any other mucous membrane, and make sure that no cream gets into an open cut. Although many of my patients get some relief from the capsaicin creams, some people find the sensation upsetting rather than soothing.

You may experience some minor skin irritation with some of these products—if a rash develops or the irritation persists, stop using the cream. Never use any of these creams in combination with heat or under a wrap or bandage.

NSAIDs

The **non-steroidal anti-inflammatory drug,** (NSAIDs) are a class of medication that relieve pain and fight inflammation, which may manifest as redness, swelling, heat, or pain. Inflammation causes pain and slows healing, so it's terrific that these drugs address that issue, as well as giving you some respite from the pain. As you'll see, they're one of the essential tools in every doctor's kit and one of the easiest forms of self-care out there. Some of them are available by prescription only, many more are available over-the-counter, with names you'd recognize immediately, like *Aleve* and *Advil*. Let me insert a quick word of warning here against too much self-medication. Always follow the dosage instructions on the package, and never take more than the suggested amount: those aren't guidelines, they're parameters. Remember, all medications have side effects. If you require any medication, even *Tylenol*, for more than a few days, you should be making your medication decisions under a doctor's supervision. Ultimately, your course of therapy may not change, but at least you'll be fully advised of the risks, and tested routinely for potential problems.

There are two different kinds of NSAIDs, COX-1 and COX-2, so called because they inhibit two different kinds of a chemical called the COX enzyme, which triggers part of the body's response to injury.

> **WARNING:** You should be very careful with NSAIDs, and take them only with your doctor's approval. This is especially true if you have a bleeding disorder, heart or kidney problem, if you're taking blood thinning medication like coumadin, or have gastrointestinal problems like ulcers. They can cause increased blood pressure, fluid retention, ulcers, and kidney damage, and some people may also be allergic.

THE COX-1s

This category of medication includes most over-the-counter anti-inflammatory medications, like aspirin, ibuprofen (*Advil*), or naproxen sodium (*Aleve*) and prescription drugs like naprosyn, voltaren, indocin, and others.

These medications, especially the over-the-counter ones, are inexpensive, readily available, and effective, so I feel comfortable under the right circumstances recommending them to my patients. These drugs may cause an upset stomach, though, so I do recommend taking them with food.

There has been some controversy surrounding the use of anti-inflammatories with knee pain and injury, since they may increase bleeding into the joint. It's my opinion that they're beneficial, since they reduce swelling and pain and thus allow movement sooner rather than later. The sooner you regain motion, the better your long-term outcome is going to be, and the faster you'll heal. So you can take them as suggested for the first couple of days after the injury or onset of pain. These can also be helpful if you're coping with chronic pain— although you shouldn't take them on a regular basis without first talking to your doctor.

THE COX-2S

A new category of drugs has recently been approved by the Food and Drug Administration called the COX-2 inhibitors, which include medications you may have seen advertised, like *Celebrex* (celecoxib), *Bextra* (valdecoxib), *Vioxx* (rofecoxib), and, in low doses, *Mobic* (meloxicam).

Because these drugs have fewer side effects and don't promote bleeding, they're better for people with gastrointestinal problems or bleeding disorders. They're not necessarily more powerful than their over-the-counter brethren, but some people do respond better to them than they do to the other drugs (the reverse is also true—I've had people throw out their expensive prescriptions in favor of good old-fashioned, over-the-counter ibuprofen).

You should take these medications according to your doctor's prescription. Here's how I like to manage my patients: we use the drug until the pain is under control. Then I ask them to start backing away from daily medication, using other pain management techniques, exercise, and modified activity, until they're taking as little medicine as they can while still maintaining their standard of living and activity level.

The downside to the COX-2s is that they're only available by prescription from your doctor, and may be more expensive as a result, but they have become a first-line prescription for inflammation and pain because they are effective with fewer side effects.

Remember: you cannot assess the strength of a medicine by the dosage. Two hundred milligrams of one medication might be as powerful as 1000 of another. Of course, in the same drug, it does make a difference.

ACETAMINOPHEN

Acetaminophen (*Tylenol*) is not an anti-inflammatory, but it does work to relieve knee pain and may be the answer if you're prevented from taking the NSAIDs for a medical reason. It is less likely to cause stomach irritation than an NSAID. Even acetaminophen has side effects if taken on a regular basis; consult with your doctor if you're taking it all the time.

STEROIDS

We've talked about your non-steroidal options, the first line of attack against knee pain, but in some cases, you may need something more powerful. If so, your doctor may inject your knee with an anti-inflammatory corticosteroid. Some of the most commonly used steroids are cortisone, methylprednisone, *Decadron*, and *Aristocort*. Injections of these drugs are most frequently used in people who have painful, unresponsive osteoarthritis.

These injections have long-lasting effects, often up to six months, although they may be less effective after frequent use. They're not without side effects, though—there's some evidence that they actually cause the degeneration of articular cartilage. Since this is what causes osteoarthritis, you and your physician will have to weigh the benefits of managing your knee pain over contributing to the advancement of your disease.

With these shots you may also experience a "steroid flare," a period of intense inflammation immediately after the shot, which can be alleviated using ice and the NSAIDs.

Oral corticosteroids are used in the treatment of rheumatoid arthritis.

NARCOTICS

Narcotic medications such as *Vicodin*, codeine, *Percoset*, and narcotic-like medications such as *Darvocet* and *Ultraset* can be effective painkillers when you're in acute pain. They can be used in combination with or independently from the NSAIDs.

The downside of narcotics is that they have the potential to be addictive. In the past you would be encouraged to take as little narcotic pain medication as possible, holding out until the pain could no longer be tolerated. We now believe that this is in fact an addictive model, and that you should take the appropriate amount to treat the pain when you feel it—and stop when you no longer do.

I hope you'll be able to use some of these strategies, either in combination with one another or independently, in order to manage your pain. Let's now take a closer look at the structure of the knee so we can understand what goes wrong when you injure it.

■ CHAPTER THREE ■

THE ANATOMY OF THE KNEE

ake a minute now—maybe for the first time ever—to think about the demands you put on your knees. Think, for instance, about the way you use your knee over the course of a normal day. You swerve to avoid a hole in the sidewalk; you kneel to plug in a computer behind a desk; you get up fast from the couch to answer the phone; you squat to pick up a penny; you bend down to pick up a toddler. So, although the knee is primarily designed to move in only one direction, it accommodates a tremendous amount of mobility and rotational ability.

And consider that almost all of your lower extremity strength, everything you need to accelerate or jump, comes from muscles that go across the knee and the hip. This means that the knee often bears up to four times our body weight, depending on the activity we're performing. For a 175-pound man, that can mean up to 700 pounds—a truly staggering load for a joint the size of your fist!

The secret to this joint's astonishing versatility and strength lies in its unique anatomy. The knee operates as a result of a complex interplay of bones, ligaments, muscles, and tendons. I happen to find this interaction an extremely elegant one, and it works beautifully most of the time. There's a lot going on, though, and the more that's going on, the more there is to go wrong.

The Parts of the Knee

The knee is the largest joint in the body. Like the fingers and the elbow, it's a hinge joint, which means that it opens and closes in one direction like a door (with a small amount of rotation), as opposed to a ball and socket joint like the hip, which allows for a large amount of rotation.

The bones surrounding the knee provide the basic structure and stability for the leg. There are four important ones in and around the knee: the *femur*, or thighbone; the *tibia* and *fibula*, which are the bones in the lower leg; and the *patella*, which is the kneecap itself. These bones are connected to each other by four major ligaments, the *cruciate ligaments*, which run through the inside of the knee, and the *collateral ligaments*, on the outside of the knee. These ligaments also provide structure and stability by restricting the range of motion of the leg. The muscles in the leg, which are some of the biggest in the body, are attached to the bone by *tendons*.

Although the thighbone is stacked on top of the bones of the lower leg, they don't grind together because they're protected by cartilage, both *meniscal*, between the femur and the tibia, and *articular*, at the ends of the bones. Cartilage isn't the knee's only form of protection: the *bursa* are small, protective sacs, often found where the tendons connect to the bones, and much of the joint is surrounded by a fluid-filled sac called the *capsule*, which is lined by sensitive tissue called the *synovium*.

With every movement, these various components work together in harmony. And yet something can go wrong with every single one of them. As we'll be returning over and over to this basic anatomy over the course of the book, let's take a closer look at these various components, and how they work together to create movement.

BONES

There are four major bones in and around the knee. These bones are called static stabilizers because they don't change in length, or stretch— their primary job is to provide structure. They are the rods around which the rest of the parts of the leg revolve.

The femur, or thighbone, extends from the pelvis to the knee and is the longest and strongest bone in the body. The two round knobs at the end of the femur are called the *condyles*—the one closest to the inside of the leg is the *medial condyle*, and the one toward the outside is the lateral condyle. The *intercondylar notch* is the space between the two condyles, and it houses one of the knee's most important ligaments, the anterior cruciate. The femur's primary job is to distribute the weight of the upper body down into the smaller bones in the lower leg.

The femur is joined to the patella, or kneecap. The patella is what's called a *sesamoid* bone, which means that it's nestled

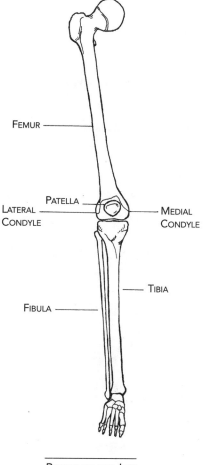

BONES OF THE LEG

inside a tendon and is designed to increase movement and decrease friction. It's a small, oval-shaped bone, which moves so your leg can move, gliding up and down in a triangle-shaped groove cut into the femur, called the *trochlear groove*.

And the patella is in turn joined to the tibia, which is commonly known as the shinbone—the second-longest bone in the body. The tibia translates the weight of the body from the femur to the foot. The fibula is the smaller bone on the outside of the leg, which helps to stabilize the knee and ankle.

As we'll see, these bones all play a crucial role in the structure, stability, and strength of the knee.

MUSCLES

The muscles connected to and surrounding the knee are considered to be dynamic stabilizers because of their ability to stretch and move. These muscles are among the largest in the body.

The *quadriceps* make up the big meaty muscle group that goes down the top of your thigh and crosses the knee in the front. The quads are composed of four separate muscles: the rectus femoris, vastus lateralis, vastus medialis, and the vastus intermedius. The quad muscles control

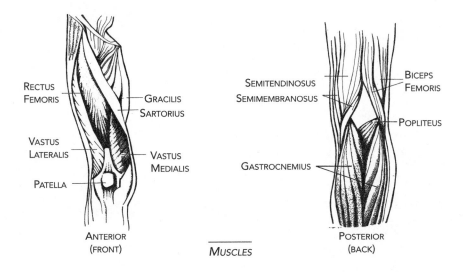

RECTUS FEMORIS

GRACILIS
SARTORIUS

VASTUS LATERALIS

VASTUS MEDIALIS

PATELLA

ANTERIOR
(FRONT)

MUSCLES

SEMITENDINOSUS
SEMIMEMBRANOSUS

GASTROCNEMIUS

BICEPS FEMORIS

POPLITEUS

POSTERIOR
(BACK)

the extension of your leg. The sartorius and gracilis muscles, or inner-thigh muscles, come from the hip to the inside of the knee. These muscles help to bring the leg inward.

Then there are the muscles at the back of your leg. The popliteus muscle is a small muscle buried deep at the back of your knee. The hamstrings are a set of big muscles at the back of your leg, running from the hip to the knee. They're really three separate muscles: the biceps femoris, the semitendinosus, and the semimembranosus, and together they're responsible for the flexion of the knee and the ability of the hip to extend.

The major calf muscle, the gastrocnemius, starts at the femur and becomes part of the Achilles tendon in the ankle. This muscle helps with flexion of the ankle but also contributes to the flexion of the knee.

The strength of the muscle groups surrounding the knee is key to knee health: the more support you're able to generate in these muscle groups, the more stable the whole mechanism is—and the less strain on the joint itself.

TENDONS

The muscles are connected to the bones by the tendons. These are really extensions of the muscles, and look like thick, white rubber bands that are stuck like glue to the ends of bones. Because of their ability to stretch, tendons are also considered to be dynamic stabilizers like the muscles they're attached to.

There are a lot of tendons in the leg—of the four quadriceps muscles each has a tendon connecting it to the patella, and one of the three major hamstring muscles has two major tendon attachments. But it is the four major tendon groups that tend to get irritated and present as knee problems: the quadriceps tendon, the patellar tendon, and the iliotibial band and the hamstring tendons.

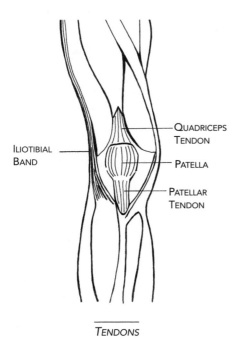

ILIOTIBIAL
BAND

QUADRICEPS
TENDON

PATELLA

PATELLAR
TENDON

TENDONS

As you can see, the quadriceps tendon attaches the quadriceps to the patella. The patellar tendon connects the patella to the tibia at a spot called the tibial tuberosity, the bony protrusion you feel right below your kneecap. This tendon connects a bone to a bone—which means that it's technically not a tendon at all, but a ligament. But since it's basically an extension of the quadriceps tendon, which is "interrupted" by the patella, it's commonly considered a tendon. The iliotibial band is a muscle-tendon combination package, and it stretches all the way from your ilium (your pelvis) to your tibia, and is a common player in knee pain. The hamstring tendons attach to the tibia and the fibula.

The tendons are prone to overuse, and when something irritates them, they can become inflamed. If that inflammation goes on long enough, you may suffer from a buildup of scar tissue in the area or a tear.

LIGAMENTS

The bones are connected to each other by four major ligaments: one on each side of the leg, and two right down the middle of the knee joint. These ligaments, considered static stabilizers because they're only capable of slight stretching, work to protect your knee from going too far out of alignment by serving as restraints in all four directions. In other words, they allow the knee to move, but not too much—an important function in preventing injury.

The two ligaments on the outsides of the joint are called the collateral ligaments: the *medial collateral ligament* (MCL) and the *lateral collateral ligament* (LCL). The MCL is on the inside of the leg, the side closest to the other leg, and connects the femur to the tibia. The LCL is on the outside of the leg and attaches the femur to the fibula. These collateral ligaments protect your knee from moving too far from side to side.

The two ligaments running through the center of the joint are the cruciate ligaments: the *anterior cruciate ligament* (ACL) in the front and the *posterior cruciate ligament* (PCL) in the back. While the MCL connects the femur to the tibia on the outside of the knee, the ACL attaches these bones on the inside of the knee. The ACL prevents the lower leg from moving too far forward. The posterior cruciate ligament (PCL) also attaches the femur to the tibia, and prevents the lower leg from moving too far back.

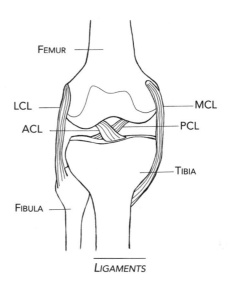

LIGAMENTS

Because the knee's motion isn't limited by a strong bony structure, like the ankle, the ligaments have a lot of work to do. And because the ligaments are charged with acting as brakes on the joint, they're particularly prone to injury. When some movement (a pivot) or some thing (a linebacker) forces the knee to do something outside of what the governing ligament can tolerate, that ligament may rip.

CARTILAGE

The bones in the knee are cushioned by cartilage. Cartilage is spongy, flexible tissue; it's the stuff your ears and the end of your nose are made of. There are many different kinds of cartilage, and there are two different kinds found in the knee: meniscal and articular.

There are two menisci in every knee: the *medial meniscus*, which is C-shaped, and the *lateral meniscus,* which is semi-circular. This cartilage is like the rubber washer you find in a kitchen faucet. It provides a cushion for the bone of the femur, preventing it from grinding up against the tibia, and providing a smooth surface so the bones can glide against each other easily when moving. The menisci also act as stabilizers for the knee, helping to distribute weight and absorb pressure and shock.

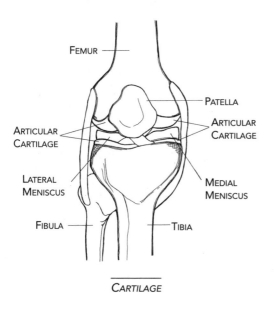

CARTILAGE

The second kind of cartilage is *articular*, which covers the ends of bones. You know the glistening, plasticky-looking stuff at the end of a chicken bone? That's articular cartilage. It protects the ends of the bones, absorbing shock, providing a cushion and a smooth surface to facilitate movement.

Cartilage takes a beating—it's load bearing, and it endures a lot of repetitive stress. It's also right in the middle of the action, so when something else gets damaged, like a ligament, the cartilage is often a secondary victim. And since it has a relatively limited ability to repair itself, it's prone to degeneration, which can cause arthritis.

BURSA

The bursa are small, fluid-filled sacs. These are very common around all the joints, and there are lots of them in the knee, especially over the spots where the tendons attach to the bones. They're designed to decrease friction across those sites.

When something irritates the bursa, they swell with fluid, which is common and can be very painful. This is called **bursitis**.

SYNOVIUM

Much of the knee is surrounded by a balloon called *the capsule*, and the lining of that capsule is called *the synovium*. The capsule is normally filled with fluid, which encourages smooth, frictionless movement and brings nutrients to the parts on the inside of the knee. When something irritates the synovium, it fills with more fluid than normal in response. This causes very painful swelling.

The *plica* is a fold in the synovial lining, a remnant from a stage of fetal development. Not everyone has one, but those who do may

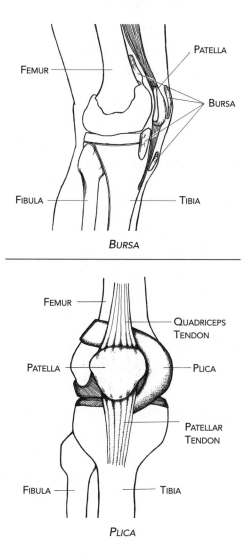

BURSA

PLICA

experience pain when the plica is irritated through overuse or injured through trauma.

How the Knee Works

Now, how do these knee parts work together? What really happens when you decide to walk from one side of the room to the other?

Most movement (except for the involuntary kind—things like your heartbeat and your reflexes) actually starts in the brain. When you decide you want to take a walk, your brain sends nerve impulses through the central nervous system, through the brain stem and the spinal cord, into all the nerves of the hip, leg, and foot. The nerves then fire the muscles, "telling" them to move in the way your brain has specified.

Muscles move in opposition to one another. When one muscle is lengthening in what's called an **eccentric contraction**, the other opposing muscle is shortening, which is called a **concentric contraction**. You can see this happening: straighten your leg in front of you, and as the hamstring at the back of your leg lengthens, you'll see the quadricep muscle at the front of your leg bunch up and tighten. Bend your leg to stretch your quad, and you'll feel your hamstring contract.

Because the muscles work in opposition to one another, when the brain calls for your leg to bend, your nerves are really sending simultaneous messages to many muscles. They're telling the hamstring muscles at the back of your leg to shorten, which means that they must also tell the quad muscles at the front of your leg to lengthen to accommodate the movement.

As the hamstring muscle shortens, it sets off a chain of reactions that results in the lifting of the lower leg: the tendons at the end of the hamstring muscle that attach to the tibia and fibula pull up on the hinge of your knee, which raises the lower leg and the foot as it bends. The cartilage provides a smooth surface, enabling the bones to glide against each other, and the ligaments act as restraints, keeping the structure intact by guiding the leg through a tolerable range of motion. As your brain sends another message—to straighten your leg this time— the whole process happens in reverse. The quad shortens, the hamstring lengthens, the hinge of the knee straightens, and the lower leg moves with it.

Plus, the whole body works on a "closed kinetic chain," which means that movement starts from the foot up. As the old song says, your leg bone's connected to the knee bone, and the knee bone's connected to the thigh bone—and to your hip and your spine. Since the whole mechanism is structurally related, if something happens to one link in the chain, the whole thing falls apart. Injuring your knee *is* different from injuring your pinkie finger: your knee is an essential cog in the wheel.

This is why knee injuries are both so common and so debilitating. The joint is prone to injury because it's such a star, and because it's so important, it can really put you out of commission when you do hurt it.

We'll refer back to these basic anatomical terms and to the mechanism that allows the knee to move over and over as we progress through the book. Let's look now at some of the factors that put your knees at risk for pain and injury, and how you can use preventive measures to offset some of that risk.

PART II

PREVENTING
KNEE INJURY

CHAPTER FOUR

WHAT PUTS
YOU AT RISK:

Biological Factors

Before we can answer the question "What can I do to protect my knees?", we have to address another one: "What is putting your knees at risk?" An injury occurs as the result of an activity and results in some restriction of your activities. It's a simple fact that certain people are at greater risk for knee pain and injury than others. That shouldn't be cause for panic. If you know what's putting you at risk for injury or re-injury, and why you're at greater risk to begin with, you can be more aggressive about taking preventive measures.

As we've discussed, the knee is a fairly vulnerable joint in all of us, simply because of where it's located and how much use it gets. When this overall vulnerability is combined with a predisposition toward knee injury, it can be a real recipe for trouble.

It goes without saying (although I'll say it anyway) that you should see a doctor if you're experiencing serious or regular knee pain as a result of any of these conditions. You can only take self-diagnosis and do-it-yourself treatment so far. But if your pain is minor and inter-mittent, the advice I've included in this section may be all you need to address these risk factors without a physician's assistance.

If it ain't broke, don't fix it. You may have one or some of the risk factors listed below, but if you're not actually experiencing knee pain as a result, you can opt to do very little (or nothing) about it, or consider taking preventive steps to avoid it developing into one.

One more thing: you don't need to sprain your bank account to stay in good knee health. I'm always in favor of proactive moves to prevent injury, but I'm conscious, as both a health care practitioner and a consumer, that you can spend thousands of dollars on "preven-tive" braces and orthotics that may not help to prevent a knee issue—and in some cases may cause further harm. Try an inexpen-sive, over-the-counter shoe insert, for example, before going to specially molded orthotics, and see what that does to help your pain. As you'll see, the best prevention measures—strengthening the muscu-lature around the knee, and staying limber—are free. I'll direct you to the programs later in this book that will help you to shore up your defenses.

Let's consider some of the things that might be increasing your risk—and what you can do to fight back.

THE RISK FACTORS

ALIGNMENT

LEG-LENGTH DISCREPANCY

LOOSE-JOINTEDNESS

GENES

GENDER

PREVIOUS INJURY

Alignment

Your natural alignment, the way the parts of the leg are positioned in relation to one another, is one of the biggest factors determining your susceptibility to knee injury. Everyone has a certain amount of variation in the way their bodies are put together, and the leg is a closed system: when one of the components in the leg is "out of alignment" it can throw the others out of whack as well. This can mean that the joint is predisposed to injury because of the extra load it carries all the time, or because it has less protection and more sensitive parts closer together. Or it can mean that you're more prone to overuse injuries or arthritis because you're wearing the knee down unevenly.

So what can you do? There *are* certain corrections we can make to your alignment through orthotics and exercise, and, in more radical cases, bracing and surgery. Let's take a closer look at how alignment affects your knee—from the ground up.

FOOT

The leg's alignment actually starts on the ground; the architecture of your foot and the way it meets the earth can have a radical effect on your knee. In fact, you can tell an awful lot about your alignment just by looking at a pair of shoes you wear often. If the wear is uneven beyond the normal pattern, you can be sure that the wear on your knee will be uneven as well.

People who are flat-footed or who have low arches tend to **overpronate**, which means that the ankle collapses inward. This makes the lower leg bones rotate inward, which increases the load carried on the inside of the knee. On the other hand, people with really high arches may **oversupinate**, which means that they tend to roll their weight onto the outside of the foot, rotating the leg bones outward and increasing the load on the outside of the knee.

If you're unsure of the status of your arch, look at the mark your foot leaves when you get out of the shower or pool. If the entire outline of your foot shows, then you have flatfeet. If the outline of the toes and ball of your foot appears to be connected to the heel by only a very thin strip, then you have high arches. A normal arch leaves a strip about half the width of the foot.

Because abnormal mechanics come into play with every step we take, they often manifest themselves in knee pain or injury, either because a badly aligned joint is more prone to injury, or simply through overuse.

For instance, people with flatfeet are often diagnosed later in life with osteoarthritis of the medial, or inside, part of the knee—in the same way that the soles of their shoes wear down faster on the inside than outside because of the way they walk or run, the inside of their knees may wear out faster than the outside does. They're also prone to iliotibial band syndrome, patellar tendinitis, and patellofemoral

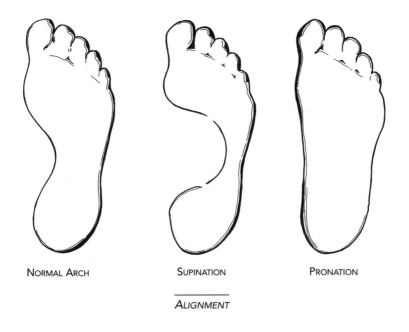

NORMAL ARCH   SUPINATION   PRONATION

ALIGNMENT

syndrome, all of which we'll discuss later in more detail. People with high arches, on the other hand, tend to have more rigid foot and ankle structures, which can make them more prone to stress fractures, tendinitis, and osteoarthritis. Addressing foot alignment issues is often a good way to deal with pain as a result of malalignment.

TIBIA

Working our way up the leg, we find the tibia, or the shinbone. In some people, instead of running straight down from the knee to the ankle, the shinbone rolls in—or out—too much. Tibial rotation is a function of the way the bone has developed, and it affects the stress load carried by the knee. Both internal and external rotation can cause tendon problems and early degenerative arthritis in the knee, because you're putting more stress on one side of the knee than the other.

KNEE

You can also have malalignment in the knee joint itself. This is seen as bowleggedness (which we call **genu varus**) and knock knees (**genu valgus**). As with any malalignment, the pressure that these particular alignment issues puts on the knee can damage the meniscal and artic-

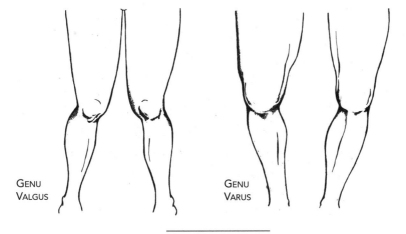

GENU VALGUS   GENU VARUS

KNEE MALALIGNMENT

ular cartilage, and either issue can cause degenerative arthritis in the knee. In bowlegged people, the damage occurs to the cartilage on the medial side (inside) of the knee; in knock-kneed people, it's the outside that suffers. Everyone has some degree of varus or valgus in their knee; neutral to a little valgus (turned out) is considered "normal," and women tend to be more knock-kneed than men.

There are also different kinds of patellar malalignment, which means that the patella, or kneecap, is either riding too low (patella baja, or patella infera) or too high (patella alta) on the thighbone, too much to the inside or the outside, or with too much of a tilt (**lateral patellar tilt and/or subluxation**). You're born with the tendency to develop patella alta; patella baja is often the result of an improperly healed surgery or trauma, which shortens the patellar tendon. These malalignments might sound like California beach towns, but no such luck. People with patella alta are more likely to suffer from knee injuries like dislocation of the knee, patellofemoral syndrome, and chondromalacia, and people with patella baja are more likely to experience tears in the quadriceps tendon and chronic knee pain.

FEMUR

The femur, or thighbone, may also twist inward (femoral anteversion) or out (femoral retroversion). Obviously, any distortion in the normal alignment of the hips and thighs pushes the knees, lower leg, and feet out of alignment as well.

You can tell if you have femoral anteversion if you find that it's easy to sit on your knees in an inverted **W**, with your lower legs drawn up beside your thighs. Femoral anteversion is more common in women, and can cause patellofemoral syndrome and chondromalacia, but happily, it's not usually associated with arthritis. Femoral retroversion, which causes toeing out, is less common.

THE Q ANGLE

The Q angle is the measure of the alignment between the pelvis, leg, and foot. To measure your Q angle, you'd draw a line between the bumpy bone right at the top of your shinbone (the tibial tubercle) straight through the center of the kneecap. That's the first side of the angle. The second side of the angle is a line from the very center of the kneecap to the front of the hipbone that sticks out right below the level of your belly button (the ASIS, short for anterior superior iliac spine). The angle created by these two lines is your Q angle.

Women tend to have greater Q angles than men because their hips are wider—a normal Q angle for a woman is between 15 and 20 degrees, and a normal Q angle for a man is between 10 and 15 degrees. As we'll discuss in later chapters, this is one of

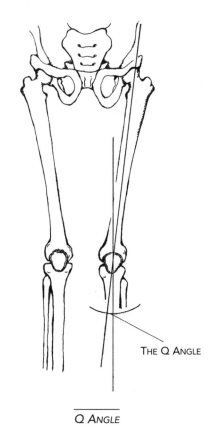

THE Q ANGLE

———

Q ANGLE

the reasons women are more prone to certain kinds of knee injuries. A large Q angle is associated with higher rates of patellar dislocation, ACL injury, patellofemoral syndrome, chondromalacia, and other knee problems.

Miserable Malalignment Syndrome

Miserable Malalignment syndrome, or Malicious Malalignment syndrome, is a classic combination of alignment issues that conspire to make those who suffer from it extremely prone to knee injury.

The syndrome is a combination of some of the alignment issues we've already discussed: femoral anteversion, knock-knees, externally rotated tibias, and flatfeet. In other words, the hips and thighs are turning in, while the lower leg is turning out. This is an interesting example of the way the body works to compensate for its own alignment issues. Here's what happens from the waist down. You naturally have femoral anteversion, so in order to make sure that the femur's head is secure in the bony socket of the pelvis, the femur has to turn in. If that alignment continued

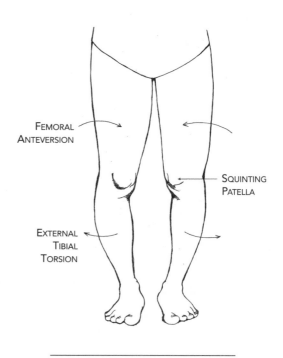

FEMORAL ANTEVERSION

SQUINTING PATELLA

EXTERNAL TIBIAL TORSION

MISERABLE MALALIGNMENT SYNDROME

all the way down the leg, the foot would be completely pigeon-toed, so the tibia compensates by rotating externally so that the foot is pointing straight ahead. That external rotation of the tibia is often accompanied by increased pronation, to accommodate the placement of the foot on the ground.

Miserable Malalignment syndrome is often found in people who have an increased Q angle, patella alta, and lateral patella tilt and/or subluxation. It's also associated with people who are very flexible, and it's much more common in women.

This syndrome is associated with all kinds of patellofemoral dysfunction. When your leg is out of alignment in this way, it puts strain on the kneecap because of the way it sits in the trochlear groove in the thighbone. When these two pieces aren't lined up as well as they need to be, they grind against each other, causing wear on the patella and irritation to the tissue surrounding it. This is a perfect recipe for chronic knee pain.

R_x

ALIGNMENT AND MISERABLE MALALIGNMENT

ORTHOTICS
Indicated for: flatfeet/high arches; Miserable Malalignment syndrome

Many of the alignment problems we've just discussed result in some distortion in the placement of the foot. Addressing this issue can alleviate your pain and prevent related knee problems as a result. For instance, flatfeet may really exacerbate the problems caused by a large Q angle, so treating that problem can be an effective preventive measure. Again, this doesn't automatically mean you have to be fitted by a specialist; inexpensive shoe inserts designed to support flatfeet and high arches are available over-the-counter at drugstores and sporting goods stores. If you have these alignment issues and suspect that they're causing persistent problems in your knees, you may want to consider being fitted for inserts by an orthotics specialist if retail inserts don't work.

EXERCISE
Indicated for all malalignment issues, especially increased Q angle; Miserable Malalignment syndrome

A program of strengthening and flexibility for the muscles around the leg is the single most effective preemptive strike you can make against knee pain.

You can also use targeted exercises to compensate for certain of these alignment issues. For both increased Q angle, lateral patellar tilt and/or subluxation, and Miserable Malalignment syndrome, you'll want to strengthen the quadriceps muscles, such as the vastus medialis (VMO), because these are the muscles that give the kneecap support. The exercises in the Knee Health Workout (see Chapter 12) will help. Miserable Malalignment Syndrome is often accompanied by tight hamstrings, so increasing flexibility in the back of the leg by doing our Stretching Workout (see Chapter 12) will also help to prevent injuries.

BRACING AND SURGERY
Indicated for severe cases of bowleggedness; knock-knees; femoral anteversion and retroversion, tibial rotation; large Q angle; patellar tilt and subluxation; Miserable Malalignment syndrome

We usually catch these really severe alignment issues in childhood, and much of the time they resolve themselves naturally. In cases where it does not, bracing or surgery may be required. In serious cases of Miserable Malalignment syndrome, knee braces can help adjust the alignment artificially. If your Q angle is abnormally large, there are also surgical solutions for people with persistent recalcitrant pain as a result of this syndrome, ranging from a relatively noninvasive arthroscopic procedure called a lateral release to a much bigger (and rarely indicated) procedure that realigns the upper part of the tibia to the patella.

There is always a danger with braces, because they add weight to the leg and change the load on the knee. With the exception of small, pull-on sleeves, wraps, and pads, do not purchase and apply your own brace; this is something that should be done only in consultation with your doctor. And don't use someone else's old brace, even if it worked for that person on a similar problem. All bodies are different, and all knee conditions are different, and this form of self-diagnosis can lead to more severe problems as easily as it can lead to recovery.

Leg-length Discrepancy

Leg-length discrepancy is another structural anomaly that can put you at risk for knee injury. Most of us are a little uneven—one leg is slightly longer than the other one. The difference can be in the tibia or the femur, or in both. Sometimes, the problem isn't in the bone at all, but the result of a muscular imbalance that makes the leg appear shorter. This is called a functional leg-length discrepancy. Most of the time, in both cases, the difference is less than half an inch, and it doesn't have an effect on the way we live.

If the difference is more than half an inch, it can make a difference in terms of your knee health, putting a greater amount of strain on the hip and the knee on one leg. It's not uncommon to see this leg-length effect in runners who always run the same way along a banked road, which artificially makes one leg longer than the other and puts an uneven load on the knees, which is why I always recommend that runners vary their routes on a regular basis.

People with significant leg-length discrepancies often experience an increase in iliotibial band syndrome and muscle/tendon inflammation.

> **R_x** **LEG-LENGTH DISCREPANCY**
>
> If you suspect that this is a problem, have your legs measured. If you have a true leg-length discrepancy, then a simple, over-the-counter insert in one shoe may fix the problem. If your leg-length discrepancy is functional, your doctor or a physical therapist can suggest exercises to correct the muscular imbalance.

Loose-jointedness

Some people are naturally extremely flexible. This is called hyperlaxity, or hyperelasticity, otherwise known as loose-jointedness. It's most commonly found in young females.

This is terrific if you're a gymnast (and it's certainly not an accident that so many hyperelastic children end up in gymnastics, which requires a terrific amount of flexibility), but it can wreak havoc on your knees. People are loose-jointed because their ligaments are looser than those in other people. As you'll remember, we require the ligaments to act as static stabilizers, restraining the leg's range of motion. If these static stabilizers aren't doing what they're supposed to do, then the dynamic stabilizers, the muscles and the tendons, have to work overtime. And if they're not up to it, the range of motion isn't controlled, which means that the kneecap can just pop out.

> **R_x** **LOOSE-JOINTEDNESS**
>
> Most of the time, the best cure for loose-jointedness is to build up the musculature around the knee so that these dynamic stabilizers can carry the extra load that's placed

on them. The General Knee Health Workout in Chapter 12 of this book has everything you need to build strong supporting muscles. This is also the one time I'm not pushing stretching as a preventive measure; people with loose joints are flexible enough without help.

Bracing can also help to restrict the range of motion. There are times when the knee is so loose that it's totally dysfunctional, and in those cases, the knee has to be surgically reconstructed.

Genes

Many of the risk factors above (like flatfeet and leg-length discrepancy), are genetic in nature, but it's also believed that your genes carry a predisposition to certain kinds of knee pain and injury, such as arthritis.

R_x GENES

Your family history doesn't give us enough information to treat you if you don't have any symptoms, but if both your parents have severe arthritis that can't be traced to previous trauma or obvious overuse, you're going to want to watch out for the first signs in yourself. Visit a doctor as soon as symptoms manifest, and I strongly encourage you to use the appropriate preventive exercises and stretches in this book before problems occur.

Eventually, gene testing will allow us to know who's predisposed to various kinds of injury and degeneration, so we can get really proactive about prevention.

Gender

Women run a greater risk of certain kinds of knee injuries than men, and there are more knee injuries in women in general. Why? We're not entirely sure, but one predisposing factor is clear: women's bodies are built differently. Their pelvises are wider and they have a biological tendency toward knee valgus (knock-knees), which changes their alignment. Women also tend to carry more body fat than men do and they have smaller muscle fibers. Their intercondylar notch is smaller. Their Q angle is wider. All these things make them more susceptible to patellofemoral pain and injury. The ACL (anterior cruciate ligament) injury is the demon that plagues women's athletics. We now think that it may be linked to estrogen receptors as well as these alignment issues, and a great deal of exciting research is taking place on other potential factors putting women at risk.

Another factor that increases women's risk of knee injury, interestingly enough, is pregnancy. When pregnant, especially in the later stages, a woman's body releases a hormone called relaxin, which loosens all the ligaments in the body in anticipation of labor. Unfortunately, her knee stabilizers are relaxing just at the moment that the woman needs them most. She is gaining weight, which is part of a healthy pregnancy but puts an extra load on the knee, and her center of gravity is also changing, which interferes with her natural balance. These things in combination mean that pregnant women must be very careful to protect their knees.

In the past, we probably would have said that men were at a higher risk for post-traumatic arthritis, the kind of arthritis you get in a joint that has been injured. In past generations, men were more active than women in both labor and sport, and therefore more prone to injury. Osteoarthritis is now between 1.5 and 4.0 times more common in women, and we're only expecting that statistic to increase. As our world has changed, the gender gap has closed—and with it, the knee health benefits of a comparatively sheltered existence. We're already seeing many more instances of post-traumatic arthritis in women, a problem that's only going to get worse because women tend to live longer than men.

Rx GENDER

Targeted strength training and flexibility, especially in the lower extremities, may help to overcome some of the factors that put women at risk. I recommend that active women, especially those with some of the other risk factors in this chapter regularly practice my General Knee Health and Stretching Workouts (see Chapter 12) regularly—even if they aren't experiencing pain. I've also included in Chapter 12 a workout that's specifically designed to help prevent ACL injury, which is a must for women of any age who participate in sports with a high incidence of those injuries, like soccer and basketball.

If you're pregnant, it's essential to maintain your trunk and lower body strength with exercises like those found in the General Knee Health Workout (but please talk to your healthcare practitioner before beginning any exercise program). Don't overstretch, and take special care to maintain your balance, especially when you're exercising.

Previous Injury

A prior knee injury does put you at higher risk for knee pain and injury in the future.

First, you run the risk of re-injury. The body has an astonishing ability to regenerate itself, but that process doesn't always happen as well as it needs to, especially if the previous injury wasn't treated appropriately or the tissue hasn't been given enough time to heal. Some knee injuries are prone to become chronic, like patellar tendinitis. And an injury may interfere with your proprioception, your body's understanding of where your limbs are in space at any given moment. This can make you more liable to fall off balance, or misjudge distance, or to come down wrong on the leg.

Second, you run the risk of compensatory injury. If the original injury hasn't healed correctly, your body will make subtle adjustments to protect the area. This can cause you to favor the other leg, or the other side of the injured leg, or a different muscle group altogether than the one weakened by the injury. This forces your body out of its natural alignment, and when your body isn't working the way it's designed to work, it's more prone to injury.

As we've discussed, many injuries automatically put you at higher risk for post-traumatic arthritis. The fact that you have had a previous injury alters the internal framework of the knee and can start the process that leads to the development of osteoarthritis. Any kind of injury that decreases the knee's natural ability to protect itself, like an ACL injury, a fracture, or a surgically removed meniscus, increases that risk.

R_x PREVIOUS INJURY

The best way to manage this risk is to *make sure that the original injury is treated appropriately and heals normally.* Get the right diagnosis, treatment, and post-injury rehab, which will improve your proprioception and strength. Bracing may add support to the injured leg, but it may also add an additional load, so that's something to discuss carefully with your doctor.

It's especially important to give the previous injury enough time to heal, so you're not working with partially damaged tissue. Concentrate on rebuilding the supporting musculature, and promoting flexibility, so that your knee has the best support possible. You'll find both a general stretching program and a knee health workout, as well as injury-specific workouts, in Chapter 12. A life-long exercise and stretching program is the only way to ensure that you are doing everything possible to prevent re-injury of your knee, so please, if you've had any sort of knee injury at all, take these exercises seriously and perform them regularly—even if you are no longer experiencing any pain or discomfort.

REMEMBER: You may have to alter your lifestyle slightly after the injury has healed. This doesn't mean you have to give up your sport, just that you have to be realistic about what you can and can't do. You don't have to give up skiing, but you may not be able to attack moguls the way you used to. You don't have to give up tennis, but you may have to put the racquet down after two sets instead of the three you used to play. Listen to your knee! Use pain as your guide, and stop the activity immediately if you feel any discomfort—playing through pain after an injury will only increase your recovery time.

CHAPTER FIVE

WHAT PUTS YOU AT RISK:

Controllable Factors

I n this chapter, we'll explore some of the things *in your control* that may be putting you at risk, complete with some constructive, proactive advice as to how you can master these risk factors and prevent injury as a result.

As you read on, you'll notice that one central concept keeps emerging: balance. Knee health is all about maintaining a balance between the knee and the stresses upon it, and a lack of balance is one of the chief reasons we're facing this knee crisis. I'd like you to think about this concept of striking a balance in your own life between work and play, between activity and inactivity, and between an injured and noninjured state, keeping these guidelines in mind:

- Lose Excess Weight
- Improve Your Conditioning
- Improve Your Flexibility
- Improve Your Bone Fitness

• Know Your Body's Cycles

• Hydrate Yourself

Lose Excess Weight

According to the American Obesity Association, approximately 127 million Americans are overweight, 60 million are obese, and 9 million are seriously obese. And those numbers are growing, especially among children.

This has serious consequences on our knee health. Overweight people suffer from more knee injuries. Like a building or a bridge, your body is designed to carry a certain load. When you exceed that load, you're forcing your body to do something it's not designed to do, and that's going to compromise your foundation. So maintaining your ideal weight isn't about looking like someone in a magazine, it's about making sure that you're not putting undue stress on your body by overloading it.

If you're not sure if you're overweight, we've provided you with a way to find out in the "Am I Overweight?" box.

R_X I always recommend that patients can avoid further knee injury by losing their excess body fat. You don't have to lose huge amounts of weight to see a difference. Even five or ten pounds can relieve some of the stress on your joints. The best way to lose weight is burn more calories than you take in. Eat a sensible, balanced diet, rich in protein, fruits, and vegetables. If you combine this with an exercise program, you will lose weight. For help, read the weight loss tips on pages 53-55.

AM I OVERWEIGHT?

Carrying excess body weight is one of the worst things you can do for your knees. It's this simple: lose the weight, and your knee health will improve.

But how do you know if you're overweight? The Body Mass Index (BMI) is a good way to tell if you're carrying too much weight for your frame. All you have to know is how tall you are and how much you weigh.

If your BMI is:

Below 18.5: You're underweight.
Between 18.5 and 24.5: You're an appropriate weight.
Between 25 and 29.9: You're overweight.
30+: You're considered obese.

On the following chart, find your height on the left-hand axis and your body weight (in pounds) in the body of the chart. Your BMI will be the number at the top of the column.

Note: While Body Mass Index is widely used, it is a blunt instrument. A very muscular person may weigh a lot for their frame, even though they're not really "overweight." And your BMI is not a test of your conditioning. You might be skinny and flabby, with no muscle tone—a situation that sets you up for a whole other set of knee problems. If your BMI is 25 or above, you have a little work to do—but don't be overwhelmed! Even a five or ten pound weight loss can make a difference.

FIND YOUR HEIGHT ON THE LEFT-HAND AXIS AND YOUR BODY WEIGHT (IN POUNDS) IN THE BODY OF THE CHART. YOUR BMI WILL BE THE NUMBER AT THE TOP OF THE COLUMN.

BMI	19	20	21	22	23	24	25	26	27	28	29	30	31	32	33	34	35
Height [in]									Weight [lbs]								
58	91	96	100	105	110	115	119	124	129	134	138	143	148	153	158	162	167
59	94	99	104	109	114	119	124	128	133	138	143	148	153	158	163	168	173
60	97	102	107	112	118	123	128	133	138	143	148	153	158	163	168	174	179
61	100	106	111	116	122	127	132	137	143	148	153	158	164	169	174	180	185
62	104	109	115	120	126	131	136	142	147	153	158	164	169	175	180	186	191
63	107	113	118	124	130	135	141	146	152	158	163	169	175	180	186	191	197
64	110	116	122	128	134	140	145	151	157	163	169	174	180	186	192	197	204
65	114	120	126	132	138	144	150	156	162	168	174	180	186	192	198	204	210
66	118	124	130	136	142	148	155	161	167	173	179	186	192	198	204	210	216
67	121	127	134	140	146	153	159	166	172	178	185	191	198	204	211	217	223
68	125	131	138	144	151	158	164	171	177	184	190	197	203	210	216	223	230
69	128	135	142	149	155	162	169	176	182	189	196	203	209	216	223	230	236
70	132	139	146	153	160	167	174	181	188	195	202	209	216	222	229	236	243
71	136	143	150	157	165	172	179	186	193	200	208	215	222	229	236	243	250
72	140	147	154	162	169	177	184	191	199	206	213	221	228	235	242	250	258
73	144	151	159	166	174	182	189	197	204	212	219	227	235	242	250	257	265
74	148	155	163	171	179	186	194	202	210	218	225	233	241	249	256	264	272
75	152	160	168	176	184	192	200	208	216	224	232	240	248	256	264	272	279
76	156	164	172	180	189	197	205	213	221	230	238	246	254	263	271	279	287

Lose Weight—and Keep It Off

If your Body Mass Index is over 26, you need to lose weight for the sake of your knees—and your back, and your ankles, and your heart, and your kidneys.

Maintaining an appropriate weight is one of the best things you can do for your overall health. Contrary to popular belief, there's no miraculous weight loss cure—but it's also not an impossible task.

In my experience, the best way to lose weight and keep it off, or to maintain a healthy weight is to combine a well-balanced diet with frequent exercise. Here are some of the tips I've picked up over the years:

Don't drink your calories. Soda, alcoholic beverages, so-called energy drinks are mostly sources of sugar and calories. Choose water instead, and you can eat your meals instead of taking them through a straw.

Choose your protein well. Chicken is a better choice than red meat; white meat is a better choice than dark meat and if you leave the skin off, you eliminate tons of calories and fat. Fish is always a good choice, not just because it's low in calories and the bad fats, but because dark-fleshed cold-water fish like salmon and mackerel are rich in omega-3 fatty acids, which are good for your joints.

Graze. If you let yourself get too hungry between meals, you're going to sit down and inhale a giant meal. It's sometimes better to eat a healthy snack, or a series of small meals over the course of the day. Turn your three squares a day into six mini-meals, in other words.

Eat plentifully. If the primary focus of your diet is fruits and vegetables and low-fat protein, then you don't have to go hungry. It's the calorie-rich foods—fast food, red meat, desserts—that pack on the pounds. By all means, help yourself to seconds on the green beans; you don't have to go hungry to lose weight, and you'll be more likely to stick with the program if you're satisfied.

Exercise portion control. Portion control is out of control! We routinely pile our plates with two to four times the amount of food we really need. If you start reading the recommended portion sizes on food labels, I bet you'll be shocked by what you find. A recommended serving of meat is 3 to 4 ounces—the size of a deck of cards. The recommended serving for cheese is 1 ounce—a 1 x 1 inch cube. A cup of cooked pasta—a serving the size of your fist—is ample. Make up the difference in salad and vegetables.

Cut your added fats. Many of the calories we consume are the "invisible" ones—the butter we slather on our bread while we're waiting for the appetizers to arrive, the oil we use to start a stir-fry or to make a salad dressing. The only problem is that they're not invisible to your metabolism. Cut added fats whenever possible, and you'll notice a big difference in your spare tire.

Don't rush. It takes about twenty minutes for the chemical that tells your brain you're full to kick in. If you eat slowly, that chemical will activate itself—before you've eaten three days' worth of calories.

Keep a food log. In the same way that keeping an exercise log can make you conscious of how many miles you've run and how you felt while you were doing it, a food log can keep you on top of the amount and types of food you consume. Americans are lucky because food is plentiful and cheap, but it also means that we're not always conscious of what we're eating. When you grab a handful of candy out of that bowl in the reception area every time you pass it, or finish your toddler's leftovers, you are consuming calories that you will eventually either have to burn or carry around with you. Writing down everything you eat will alert you to your trouble areas and provide a lot of incentive for keeping your hands in your pockets.

Move it and lose it. Exercise, in combination with a healthy diet, is one of the best ways to lose weight. First of all, studies have shown that if you lose weight through exercise and a healthy diet, you'll be more likely to keep it off than if you lost it through exercise alone. Exercise burns calories, the first order of business for someone looking to lose weight. And it raises your metabolism, so that you continue to burn more calories over the course of the day than you would if you'd been idle. It helps you to build muscle, which makes your body a more efficient calorie-burning machine, and it makes you feel more active and confident.

Increasing the amount of exercise you get isn't hard to do. If you're mostly inactive right now, then focus on increasing "your activities of daily living" or the amount of exercise you get over the course of an ordinary day. Leave your car at the back of the parking lot instead of taking the spot right in front of the store. Take the stairs at your office— in the morning, at the end of the day, and to and from lunch. If your office is on the eleventh floor, get off at nine and walk up the rest of the way—and at eight next week, and seven the week after. Make yourself the official family dog-walker, and gradually increase the amount of time you spend walking him after dinner from ten to twenty to thirty minutes. You'll be pleased by your weight loss—and by the way your knees will feel as a result (unless, of course, all of the added stairs begin to give you knee pain). If you're already working out, then you may need to retool the effectiveness of your workout. You need to get your heart rate up, and work just a little bit harder every day than you did the day before to see weight-loss results.

Improve Your Conditioning

The overall condition you're in has a direct impact on your knee health. If you're in poor condition, meaning you have very little strength in your legs and your torso, you put yourself at high risk from knee injury by performing the simple activities of daily life. If there's no musculature supporting the knee, then simply getting up off the couch or walking to the corner store can put a tremendous amount of pressure on the knee. It's muscle that pulls and pushes the knee into position. If the muscles surrounding the knees are weak, then there's nothing helping the knee to do the job you're asking of it.

If you're in poor condition, whether as the result of an injury or just taking time off, you're at higher risk for injury. The best way to counter that risk is to get into shape, slowly and intelligently.

When we're conditioning, recovering, or just becoming more active, it's easy to forget the muscles surrounding the knee in favor of the more obvious arm and leg muscles. It is also easy to overlook the trunk: the abs, the hips, the buttocks, and the lower back. This is your core, your center—like the trunk of a tree, it's the source of the root system and the support structure for everything above it. All your strength, stability, and balance comes from your midsection; if it's weak, then it can't sustain the rest of the body. And yet it's often neglected.

Unfortunately, we tend to train what we see in the mirror or the muscles we need for our sports, neglecting the supporting players, like the trunk and the hip girdle, although they're essential for every activity we do when we're erect, including walking, running, and jumping. If you're starting a conditioning routine or, even more important, feeling some discomfort when walking, running, or training, pay close attention to the muscles you're ignoring: they may be the source of your problem. If you're not training at all, you need to remember, as I'll say over and over again, that muscle strength and flexibility are two of the most important factors in preventing knee injury.

Even if you're in good shape, you could still be at risk. I always warn active people to watch out for *evenly distributed strength*. It's common to train unevenly, meaning that we concentrate more on the muscles in the front of the body than we do on the ones in the back, or the muscles on the outside as opposed to the ones on the inside. As you'll see, these discrepancies can cause real problems. Your dominant leg (the one you kick with), may be significantly stronger than your nondominant leg. If so, your weaker leg is more vulnerable to injury—and that weakness could be causing you to over-rely on your stronger leg, leaving that one susceptible as well.

Conditioning is relative—even within a leg. I had a high-level amateur cyclist come in for a second opinion on his patellofemoral knee pain. "The other doctor told me I had to improve my quad strength," he said, looking down at his massively muscular thigh in disbelief.

Believe it or not, that other doctor was right. Of course, the problem wasn't a lack of overall muscle in his already monstrous, incredibly strong quads. But he did need to strengthen his medial quads in relation to his lateral quads—the inside of his leg in relation to the outside. His inner thighs were impressive, but because of his serious bicycling his outer thighs were even more impressive, and when the two opposing muscle groups were engaged around his patella, the bigger muscles on the outside were firing faster and stronger, dragging his kneecap over to their side. So the issue wasn't a lack of strength, but an imbalance in conditioning.

As you'll see, the whole issue of balance and timing is an essential piece in the knee injury puzzle, especially when we're talking about people in terrific shape, like this cyclist. Strength in and of itself isn't the only conditioning issue you need to be aware of. Relative strength and conditioning—from side to side, and even between muscle groups in the same leg—is essential as well because the speed at which the muscle fires relative to the rest of the leg impacts movement and performance.

Rx My General Knee Health Workout (see Chapter 12) strengthens all the supporting muscle groups in the leg and is your best preemptive strike against knee pain. This workout contains a number of exercises specifically designed to improve your muscle timing and balance as well as muscle strength. Doing it regularly will help you eliminate any firing discrepancies among your muscles.

Improve Your Flexibility

There has been much discussion in the sports medicine community as to whether stretching reduces injury, and the evidence is mixed. At the end of the day, I'm one of the people who believes that one way to buttress yourself against knee injury is to stay flexible. In general, the greater your range of motion, the better you're able to distribute forces across the knee. And many of the knee injuries we'll be covering in this book are the direct result of tight muscles feeding into the knee.

You have to watch out for unevenly distributed flexibility in the same way you have to watch out for unevenly distributed strength. If you've ever done yoga, you won't be surprised to learn that most people are considerably more flexible on one side than on the other. It may take a little work, but you can even yourself out.

R_X STRETCH!

The Stretching Workout in Chapter 12 is an excellent introduction to some ways you can increase the flexibility of the muscles around the knee. I recommend that my patients stretch at the beginning and end of every workout, and on a regular basis, as part of a physically active day.

Improve Your Bone Fitness

In my experience, most people forget that bone fitness is as important as cardiovascular or muscular fitness—doing what you can to keep your bones fit is a important step in avoiding injury.

Bone is a living substance. It renews itself the same way your skin does, and that renewal process is stimulated by stress. A little stress is a good thing, because it encourages the bone to rebuild itself and makes it stronger. But too much stress at once is a bad thing, because you're overloading the system and can't produce new bone as fast as you need it.

So, if you've never run before and start running a lot, you're putting yourself at risk for stress fracture. If you've become more active (or differently active, as I'll explain later) and you're feeling pain in your bones, that's a first sign that you're manifesting some weakness there. If you ignore that pain and run through it, you're going to develop a stress fracture, and you're going to be off your feet for a while. If you listen to the pain, give it a little rest until it feels better and then concentrate on cross-training and building your strength gradually, the bone will grow to accommodate the added stresses, and you'll ultimately be rewarded with a stronger bone.

It pays to know where you are on the bone-strength continuum. Women reach peak bone strength earlier than men, but they start losing it earlier, and it drops precipitously after menopause.

You also have to factor in your bone-strength history. Your bone strength decreases as you age, thus age is a factor. It's partially genetically determined. But what you've been doing all those years counts, too. If you've been running or doing some other weight-bearing exercise for forty years, your bones are going to be stronger than someone's who hasn't, and your bones will probably respond better to additional stresses.

R$_x$ Ease into activity gradually, introducing your bones to new stresses over time. Listen carefully if you experience any pain in your bones. Everyone, especially women over fifteen years old, should make sure they're getting 1500 mg of calcium, and 400 I.U. of vitamin D a day. If you live in someplace like the North Pole, or anywhere that you're not guaranteed a minimal amount of sunlight every day, consider supplementing your diet with even more Vitamin D.

Know Your Body's Cycles

One of the emerging issues in sports medicine is the correlation between when you work out and when you get injured and though no hard and fast conclusions have been drawn, it's something that people should take into consideration when calibrating their risk. When you train at the same time every day, you're training your brain and body to be ready for that activity at that time—and your assumptions about your performance are based on the conditions of that time of day. But it might be a little hotter during an afternoon game than when you usually practice in the morning, or your body may require a little more warming up in the morning than it does when you hit the gym after work; thus assumptions may be based on false criteria.

This doesn't necessarily mean that you have to fall into a lockstep of working out at the same time every day—it just means that you have to take these factors into consideration. If it's hotter in the afternoon, drink more water and be careful to get rest between innings. If you're a bit creaky because you just got up, extend your initial stretching period for an extra five minutes and make sure your warm-up is adequate. Also consider working out at different times of the day. However, if you are training for competition that occurs in the afternoon, do train in the afternoon.

Although this formula pertains mostly to active people, there's a bigger lesson to be learned here: pay attention to what your body is telling you. Even if you're just walking the mall, listen to your body and take a time out if that's what it's asking for. You may be more tired one day than usual, simply because of the way you slept, the food you ate, the impact of the stresses in your life. If your body needs rest, give it rest.

R$_x$ Everyone has natural cycles, and you must pay close attention to them. If you're a business traveler who travels across time zones and runs on the treadmill in your hotels, know that your brain may still be on home time, and this may mean that you're not at your optimum level when you're actually working out.

Hydrate Yourself

Keeping yourself properly hydrated is a very important step in preventing injury, but it often falls to the bottom of the list of priorities. Water is a key component in proper muscle contraction, and if your muscles aren't contracting efficiently, you'll feel weak and be subject to cramping and at much higher risk for injury.

R$_x$ Drink water every day. Drink more if you're in a hot or humid climate, and think about adding salt to your diet. Drink a 20-ounce bottle of water every hour and a half that you're working out or being physically active, even when swimming. If working out for several hours at a time, get a sports-electrolyte drink. Increase your intake a) if engaging in very strenuous activity, b) live at (or have traveled to) a high altitude, or c) the temperature and humidity are high. Remember: it's not enough to buy a bottle of water—you have to drink it!

Go Low Impact!

A knee problem—even a serious one—isn't an excuse not to exercise. In fact, the opposite is true: it makes regular exercise more important than ever. Many of the knee injuries I see are actually the result of underuse, muscles that have become atrophied to the point where a simple activity like running for the bus can overtax the structures of the knee. Being overweight significantly increases the load you're putting on your knees. Although aerobic endurance might not seem like it has much to do with knee health, your overall condition does affect the way your joints respond to stress and injury.

The key is to find an activity that doesn't hurt or make your injury worse. We know that some sports, such as running, skiing, soccer, and basketball, are hard on the knees. There are certainly ways that those sports can be modified to make them a little more knee-friendly, but they do put stress on the joint and may not be the right choice for every knee. If you're just starting an exercise program, if you're just coming back from an injury, or have other physical limitations, you'll probably want to stick with **low-impact exercise.** When you jump up and down, you put a lot of stress on your joints. Low-impact exercise enables you to build muscle and get your heart rate up without putting that stress on the knees.

SWIMMING

By far, swimming is the best low-impact exercise out there. Because your body is totally cushioned by the water, there's no stress at all on the joints. Lap swimming is a very efficient way to work out; swimming works nearly every muscle in the body, and it's certainly an effective aerobic workout. While you swim, you can also focus your attention on different parts of your body. A kickboard is a piece of foam rubber that you hold with your hands while you kick your legs; there are also foam buoys that you hold between your knees so you can work exclusively on your arms and give your knees a break.

Note: If you have knee problems, avoid the whip kick done with the breaststroke.

AQUATIC THERAPY

In the course of their rehabilitation, many of my patients have discovered aquatic therapy, and they've stuck with it long after the injury has healed. There are many variations on this, but any exercises done in a warm pool qualify. The water provides resistance (and a much more even and joint-friendly resistance than you'll find in a weight room) and enough buoyancy to make movement easy. The warmth of the pool helps crampy muscles to relax, and combats soreness. Walking in the shallow end can be effective exercise, and try doing parts of your physical therapy protocol there, too.

ELLIPTICAL TRAINERS

If you're hooked on the treadmill or the stairmaster at the gym, but find that they're murder on your knees, elliptical trainer machines provide a terrific low-impact alternative.

PILATES

Pilates, an exercise system developed in the 1920s by Joseph Pilates, uses a series of mat, table, and standing exercises to focus on improving flexibility and strength, with a lot of emphasis on the core body: the spine and lower back, the hips, and the abdominals. These muscles support the knee and are often overlooked in training and rehab, so this method can be helpful for those who suffer from knee pain.

WALKING

Walking is a good way to get started if you're out of shape, or in cardiac rehab. It's something you can do outside or on a treadmill. You can also do it anywhere and anytime, so everyone can incorporate it into their daily activities without difficulty.

CYCLING

There are many different kinds of bicycles: mountain bikes, road cycles, stationary bikes at the gym. Spinning classes, aerobic classes done on the stationary bike, are popular, and are terrific exercise. If cycling bothers your knee, see if your gym has a recumbent bike, which can take some pressure off those areas, or an arm ergometer, where you turn stationary bike pedals with your arms.

STRENGTH TRAINING

People often associate resistance training or weight training with body-building. They don't realize that they can get their heart rate up doing certain kinds of strength training with resistance. If exercises are done correctly, they can be a good workout for the joints and the bones as well. In a similar vein, total-body-conditioning classes, popular at many gyms, use fairly light weights (or just the body as resistance) as you move quickly through a series of exercises for the lower body, upper body, and abdominals. The heart rate stays up, and the exercises tone your muscles.

MODIFY AN EXISTING WORKOUT:

If you're an aerobics fan, it's possible to get a good low-impact workout in a high-impact class with just a few modifications. A rule of thumb: an exercise is low impact if you have one foot on the ground at all times. So instead of doing a jumping jack, you move your arms over your head the way you would normally, but move one leg out to the side at a time instead of hopping out with both. Most aerobics exercises can be modified in this way.

> Note: if you suffer from arthritis or are concerned about bone loss, you should spend at least a few of your weekly workouts on weight-bearing exercise, which helps to build bone.

CHAPTER SIX

THE IMPORTANCE OF PROPER TRAINING IN PREVENTING KNEE INJURY

The first step in keeping your knees safe from injury is making sure that they're up for the job you're asking them to do, and fitness training done properly is your opportunity to prepare your body for the demands your activity requires. Training improperly not only robs you of that opportunity, it actually jeopardizes your efforts.

Be honest about your current level of fitness. If you haven't been exercising at all, for instance, you may want to start with a half-hour walk each day before moving up to jogging. If you've had chronic joint pain before, perhaps you'd be better off sticking with a low-impact option until you know what your knees can take. If you're a weekend warrior, don't jump from running five miles to running a marathon.

No matter what your current level of fitness or activity, these basic training principles will help to protect you from injury.

— Build your training slowly.

— Train for your activity.

— Train in phases.

— Cross-train.

— Use the proper equipment correctly.

— Play by the rules.

— Consider additional instruction.

— Warm up, cool down, and stretch.

— Let your body recover.

Build Your Training Slowly

Most overuse injuries are the result of people doing too much, too fast, and/or too often. *If you don't train properly and carefully ease yourself into intense activity, you will get hurt.*

A patient came limping into my office after an impromptu Thanksgiving Day game of touch football with his sons. "I played ball in college," he told me, astonished that his body had betrayed him. Unfortunately, the conditioning he did twenty-five years ago wasn't protecting him from injury now. You can't just throw yourself into activity without preparing your body—or paying the price.

Even if you're in good shape, be careful not to have unrealistic expectations for your body, and don't do more than your body can handle. I see tons of patients who have injured themselves on a skiing and hiking vacation, and the story is always the same: they went mountain climbing and overdid it, they went skiing and overdid it. Windsurfing, cycling, hiking, salsa dancing—you name it, they've overdone it. Invariably, these are "fit" people, people in good shape—but not in the kind of shape they needed to be in to perform the activity they did at the intensity they did it at. Working out at the gym three or four times a week simply isn't adequate preparation for biking the Pyrenees.

Avoid making leaps in your conditioning program. Obviously, to see improvement, you have to push yourself a little past what you're accustomed to doing, but there's a difference between slowly and gradually increasing your endurance and strength, and throwing yourself headlong into severe activity. If you're planning a period of intense activity, such as a vacation, or really committing for the first time to getting fit, give yourself plenty of time to get ready.

Don't let your competitive spirit (or your buddies) goad you into working out past what your body can realistically handle. Trust me, you'll look more foolish if you end up on crutches than if you listen to your body and slow down before you get hurt.

And if you're coming back from an injury, be patient! This is a difficult pill to swallow, especially if you're accustomed to an active lifestyle and are anxious to resume your activity. If you go back to your previous level of activity before you have regained your full range of motion, strength, balance, and flexibility, you run a tremendous risk of hurting yourself again.

Train for Your Activity

You use different muscles when you swim than when you run, walk, or cycle. So, especially if you're planning a period of intense activity, it's important to train for your activity. You have to train the specific muscles you'll be using for your activity.

Train in Phases

The concept of training differently to match different phases of performance has been around since the 1960s. It's most often used in the context of high-level athletics: a football player who maintains conditioning in the off-season, starts to build muscle as the season begins, trains specifically for competitive events, and then eases himself into the post-season.

Professional athletes call this training in *periods*, or phases which correspond to the demands they're making on their bodies. If you're training for a big event, it means your level of activity is not the same year-round, and you'll need to take this into account when you're planning phases of your training and trying to prevent or deal with knee pain.

This is applicable even if you're just thinking about picking up a tennis racket for the first time since high school. This is an activity that you have to train for by getting your body into "in-season" shape. *In all cases, look realistically at your fitness plans and goals over the next few months, and organize your training schedule accordingly.* This could be the key to keeping you from experiencing knee pain, or it may be the solution to your chronic aches. There's a condition called "spring knee," an overuse injury we see in cyclists who get carried away and do too much riding as soon as the weather gets warm.

The components that you should take into consideration when you're working up to new activities, trying to sustain new activities, or organizing your training schedule without knee pain are volume (how much you do); intensity (how hard you work); frequency (how often you do it); specificity (what parts of the body you work); and recovery (how—and for how long—you let the body rest).

I recommend to all of my patients that they keep a workout journal that documents these training factors and notes how they felt while they were doing their various workouts. These journals can be a valuable tool when we're trying to figure out how your injury started, what's making it worse, and what makes it feel better.

A runner's journal might look like this:

DATE: *4/22*
_____

TIME: *1 hour*
_____

RUN MILES: *5*
_____

HILLS: *Yes*
_____

KNEE NOTES: *A little pain going downhill, no pain*

after activity
_____

_____

GENERAL NOTES: *New sneakers*: (brand name, style #, $)
_____

_____

And if your workout is the same year-round, that's another thing to take into consideration. If you swim indoors when it gets colder outside, run the same amount in the winter as you do in the summer, or travel in the summer so you can still hit the slopes, then you have to think about your own phases a little differently: in fact, you're "in-season" all year. That means you have to keep up "in-season" strength and flexibility training all-year-round as well.

CROSS-TRAIN

Your body adapts to the work you give it. If you run ten miles four times a week for a year, you'll notice it getting easier. This is partially because you're in better shape than you were when you started, but it's also because your body has "learned" to do the activity, and it takes less work than it once did. In order to continue to see an improvement, you'll have to shake up your routine.

There's an injury-prevention concept at work here, too. It's important to train for your sport, but not to the exclusion of other muscle groups. Remember, **the strength and flexibility you have in your ankles, hips, back, and trunk have a direct relationship to your knee**. Often, people concentrate on one area of their bodies at the expense of the others. For instance, it's not unusual for long-distance runners to neglect their abdominal and back muscles—even though those muscles can have a serious impact on both their performance and the stability of their knees.

One way to address this problem is to cross-train. Alternate running with days on the stairmaster or in the pool, and add some weight training to build the muscles that support your activity. Cross-training is a good way to improve your performance and combat boredom as you strengthen your entire body.

USE THE PROPER EQUIPMENT CORRECTLY

All activities require equipment, even if it's just footwear and the surface you're playing on. It's essential that your gear be appropriate, well maintained, properly sized by a professional, and that you know how to use it. We'll discuss what to watch out for when we talk about equipment for specific activities, but there are some general guidelines:

Proper equipment. Whatever your activity, make sure that you're properly outfitted. For instance, taking a walking stick on your hike can help to distribute the stress loads on your knees. While you don't have to buy every gadget and doodad on the market, it's important to keep your equipment current.

Footwear. Foot alignment issues are often the culprit behind knee pain, so your choice of footwear has real impact on the knee, especially if your sport is high-impact, like basketball, tennis, or running. Here are tips for choosing the right shoe:

— Make sure you're using the right footwear for your activity: basketball sneakers on the courts, running shoes to jog.

— Go shoe shopping late in the day. Your feet swell and stretch out over the course of the day, so if you go later, you'll get a better fit.

— Bring or wear the socks you plan to train in, and put them on when you're trying on shoes, as this will affect shoe fit. If you plan to wear orthotics, bring those as well.

Know what kind of foot you have. If your feet are wide, stick with the sneaker brands that carry widths. Go to a store that specializes in athletic shoes and talk to someone who knows how the different brands fit before you buy. (Asics run narrow, for instance, and are great for people who have a problem getting other sneakers secure around their foot.)

In the "Alignment" section of Chapter 3, I give guidelines for determining whether or not you have a flat or high-arched foot. Many athletic shoes today are marketing as "anti-pronating," which is a tremendous help to people who pronate, or have flat feet. If you have high arches, you want to look for a shoe that provides you with cushioning and shock absorption.

If you look at your athletic shoes right now, you'll probably see that a number of colored bands of foam make up the sole. A rule of thumb: the darker the foam color on a sneaker, the more rigid it is. Someone with very high arches would want bands of white (or a light color) all around the outside of the shoe, combined with a cushioned insole.

Stay away from unsupportive fabrics for the upper. There was a trend toward spandex uppers a little while ago, and while these made for spectacularly lightweight shoes, they didn't provide the kind of support an athlete needs on the inside and the outside of the foot. When that support isn't there, you lose shock absorption as well.

Replace your worn shoes when necessary. I recommend that runners replace their shoes every 250 to 400 miles. If you have high arches, I recommend that you replace them more often, in the 250- to 275-mile range.

PLAY BY THE RULES

Know the rules of the game you're playing, know where you're supposed to be, and where your teammates and opponents are supposed to be.

A surprising amount of the trauma injuries I see are the result of an accidental collision: someone was in the wrong place on the field at the wrong time and didn't have a clear idea of where the other players were. If you've never played Ultimate Frisbee before, don't be afraid to ask about the rules and hang back a bit until you understand the game.

Of course, contact sports are contact sports so I encourage you, especially if you play team sports, to stay actively aware of the other players' positions on the field, the same way you'd be aware of other cars on the road.

CONSIDER ADDITIONAL INSTRUCTION

It's never a bad idea to get additional instruction in your activity, even if you're proficient in it. Anyone who has lifted weights knows that you can waste a lot of time doing something wrong—and sometimes the margin of error is something as simple and seemingly minor as the positioning of your hand or the speed at which you do something. Remember, even the pros have coaches. Professional training—even just a lesson or two—is an excellent way to take your performance to the next level and can be an important injury prevention measure as well, especially if you specifically ask your instructor to tell you if he or she sees you doing something that puts you at risk.

WARM UP, COOL DOWN, AND STRETCH

No matter what kind of condition you're in, you should start your workout with a warm-up period, and end it with a cool-down. This doesn't have to be anything more intense and involved than a short, brisk walk to get your heart rate up combined with some gentle movements to loosen up the joints.

In an ideal scenario, you'd get your muscles warmed up, stretch, perform your activity, stretch, and then cool down. In Chapter 12, I've provided a stretching routine that is perfect for this because it hits all the major muscle groups in a short amount of time.

Warming up increases the range of motion you enjoy in your joints and raises the muscle temperature around the joints, which increases the efficiency of the muscle contraction. As we've discussed, there's some question as to whether or not stretching before activity reduces injury rates. I feel that stretching the muscle decreases the tension in the muscle–tendon unit and makes it more difficult to tear that muscle or that tendon. It feels good, it reduces next day soreness—so what do you have to lose?

WATCH OUT FOR FATIGUE

Many injuries happen when people get tired. This has been proven over and over again in studies, and it is certainly borne out anecdotally in sports medicine. People tend to get hurt in the last quarter, during the final set, on the last mile. You think, "Just one more lap," but your muscles and your brain are slower to react, and that puts you in harm's way.

When you're tempted to go back for "just one more," take a moment to realistically access your physical and mental condition. If you're really tired, then it's time to pack it in—or run the risk of an injury.

LET YOUR BODY RECOVER

Many people don't give their bodies adequate time to recover. This means that their bodies are constantly tired and weakened, and more prone to injury as a result. They are also more susceptible to infectious diseases like colds and flus, as fatigue weakens their immune systems.

I recommend that my patients take a minimum of one day a week off, with a preference of two days, and it's better if those two days aren't back to back. I also recommend that they don't work the same muscle groups in a twenty-four-hour period, so that everything has ample chance to heal and rebuild.

CHAPTER SEVEN

PLAY IT SAFER

An Activity-by-Activity
General Knee Health Guide

I
f you're an athletic person, you may be worried about knee pain and
injury. But you don't have to give up your sport to keep your knees
safe—you just have to play smarter. In this chapter, you'll notice that
we emphasize five protective conditioning features under every single
activity we talk about: **strength**, **flexibility**, **balance**, **agility**, and
timing. The best equipment in the world can't make up for poor conditioning. Keeping your body in good shape is the best prevention
measure you can take.

A NOTE ABOUT RESUMING YOUR SPORT AFTER AN INJURY

If you've suffered a knee injury, have been properly and fully treated,
and have a clean bill of health from your doctor, then there's no reason
not to resume your activity. Remember, staying in good condition is
especially important for people who have experienced knee injury,
since you're automatically at higher risk for injury. As you start to get

back into the swing of things, pay close attention to the exercise programs we recommend in this chapter to supplement your sport.

This is also a good time to take a good hard look at your training to see if you can isolate an underlying reason for your previous injury. Were you using the wrong equipment—or the right equipment improperly? Was your footwear up to snuff? Were you neglecting flexibility or strength?

You must address the issues that caused your first injury. If you don't change improper training behaviors, you're going to reinjure yourself. Be more serious next time around. It may take awhile to retrain yourself to train properly, but it's work well worth doing.

Basketball

Basketball involves lots of quick cuts, sudden stops, pivots, and jumps—all nightmares for knee health.

Common injuries: patellar tendinitis (jumper's knee), ACL sprain, patellofemoral pain, meniscal tears, patellar subluxation

How to Protect Yourself

Get the proper footwear. Wear high-topped basketball sneakers, which will provide the foot and ankle with the extra support needed to keep the knee safe. If you have flat feet, correct this with the proper shoes or a special insert.

Train properly

Agility, balance, cutting, hopping, and jumping drills are all essential tools in training your body to protect itself from injury.

Warm up. Hitting the court cold can be devastating for your knees. A proper warm-up includes running around the court at least ten times to get your muscles warm, followed by six court-long forward sprints at half speed so your body gets used to sprinting, and six backpedaling sprints at half speed to warm up muscles at the back of the body. Then do my Stretching Workout (Chapter 12), and you'll be ready to play.

Jump *right*. With a little training, you can learn to jump "right"—in a way that jeopardizes your knee least. Keep your knees aligned and underneath you at all times, instead of allowing them to splay out. As you land, use your hamstrings, not just your quads, and shift your weight from your toes to your mid-foot—like a rocking chair, and keep your knees bent. Keep moving after landing, so your body doesn't have to decelerate quite as much.

There are various exercises that assist in jumping and landing techniques I recommend to coaches, including the Henning Program in Kansas, Caraffa Program in Italy, Sportsmetric Training Program in Ohio, PEP program in California, and Ski Awareness Program in Vermont. Please note that Plyometric, or jumping exercises, should always be done under close professional supervision.

Always keep your knees bent as you land and pivot.

Strength, Flexibility, Balance, Agility, Timing

Build your eccentric strength. As we'll discuss at greater length in Chapter 12 on exercise, there are two different kinds of strength: concentric and eccentric. The "positive" part of the movement—raising your arm in a bicep curl, for instance, or jumping up—is concentric. The "negative" part of a movement—lowering your arm, or landing—is the eccentric movement. Eccentric movements require their own separate kind of strength. This is often overlooked by even the best athletes, although it's a terrific preventive measure. This is why all our workouts include eccentric training.

Build your strength ratio. Players with a good hamstring/quad strength ratio are much less likely to get injured. Increasing the strength of these two muscle groups, especially the hamstrings, will help your leg support the knee during deceleration and twisting. This is especially important for women, who are more prone to ACL injury than men. Some experts believe that this is partially because men activate their hamstrings three times more than women do when they're landing from a jump. Female hamstrings tend to be significantly weaker than their male counterparts, so strengthening this part of the body has a terrific impact on ACL injury prevention.

R_X Stretching Workout, ACL Health Workout

Cycling

Most cycling injuries are the result of overuse. Think about it—if you're cycling between 60 and 100 revolutions per minute, then your knee is performing the same task between 3,600 and 6,000 times an hour! That's a great deal of repetitive stress on the knee.

Most of the injuries I see are the result of road biking, but many of these prevention tips can and should also be applied to mountain biking—and even spin classes—as well.

Common injuries: Iliotibial band syndrome, patellofemoral pain, including plica and patellofemoral syndrome, patellar and quadriceps tendinosis; pes anserine bursitis

HOW TO PROTECT YOURSELF
Use the proper equipment

Make sure your bike is the right fit. Improper bike fit is an enormous contributing factor to knee injury. If your bike seat is too high, you're straining the hamstring tendons. If the seat is too low, you're putting yourself at risk for pain behind the patella, at or around the patella and quadriceps tendon. You should have your seat adjusted by a professional, but the quickest and easiest way to make sure you're not hurting yourself is to make sure that there's a slight (20–25 degree knee bend) when your pedal is at the bottom of the rotation. Your leg should never be completely straight. Another fast way to check your seat height is to make sure that your hips don't rock when you pedal.

The fore-aft position of your saddle is also important. Your bike shop will have a "plumb bob," a small device that you can hang off the front part of your knee while your pedal is at the three-o'clock position and

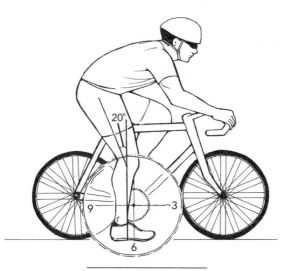

PROPER BIKE FIT/ANGLES

the soles of your feet are horizontal. The plumb should fall over the ball of the foot and the pedal spindle. Your cleat position is another important factor. If your cleat is internally rotated too far, it can cause stress to the iliotibial band. Your bike shop will be able to check your cleat alignment. Cleats with some degree of rotation are preferable to those that are fixed.

Use proper footwear. If you're planning on cycling regularly, it's worth it to invest in good shoes, or a shoe system that clips onto your pedals. Cycling shoes are relatively rigid, and can get more power out of the quads, which helps to minimize how hard the calf muscles have to work.

Correct leg-length differences. A leg-length discrepancy can put you at higher risk for knee injury. This is especially true for cyclists. If one of your legs is longer than the other one, talk to your doctor or physical therapist about putting a spacer under your cleat.

Train properly

Don't do too much too soon. The most common cycling injury I see is overtraining—doing too much too soon. There's a condition called "spring knee," which describes a pattern of overuse caused by long spring rides after a winter of undertraining. I can understand the temptation to overdo it when the sun finally comes out to stay, but if you build your strength and endurance gradually, you run less of a risk of losing your summer to an injury.

Don't build too fast. Another common overuse pattern I see is the result of someone trying to add too many miles to their workout too fast. I usually advise my patients to increase slowly, by twenty miles a week. Ease yourself into hill work a little bit at a time. It's better to do too little than too much at the beginning.

Don't ride in too low a gear. Keep very low rpms to a minimum, especially at the beginning of your training. Train in intervals, so that you're alternating periods of pressure on the knee with periods of less stress.

Maintain proper technique. When you ride behind a tired cyclist, you can actually see their form fall apart. The telltale sign is that their knees flare outward on the downstroke. As they fatigue, they're trying to engage the stronger muscle groups on the outside of the leg. Unfortunately, this isn't doing their knees any good. You must maintain a proper pedal stroke, keeping your shoulders, hip, knees, and feet in line with one another.

Quit when you're tired. As we've seen, your technique falls apart when you're tired, and that puts you at risk. Spin when it's appropriate, in order to recoup some of your energy and pump out some of the waste products. If that doesn't work, quit before you get hurt.

BUILD YOUR STRENGTH, FLEXIBILITY, BALANCE, AGILITY, TIMING

R_x *Stretching Workout, General Knee Health Workout*

Strengthen your inner leg. Because cyclists rely so heavily on their outer quadriceps muscles, they often have to strengthen and improve the firing time of the muscles at the inside of the leg to maintain a proper balance.

Football

This is a sport with a high demand for a lot of taxing cutting, jumping, pivoting, rapid starts and stops—and these are combined with contact, so football is a sport that's heavily associated with knee injury.

MCL injuries usually occur when a major force hits the outside of the leg. Because that's pretty much par for the course in football, there isn't a whole lot you can do to avoid it. But many other injuries happen as the result of a foot that's planted while the leg twists.

Common injuries: MCL, meniscal tears, ACL, PCL injuries

How to Protect Yourself
Use the proper equipment

Use proper footwear. Football-style cleats, which have long (more than half an inch) cleats, are the cause of more injuries than the shorter, soccer-style cleats, because shorter cleats don't dig into the playing surface as much, thus the foot is more mobile and available to turn with the leg.

Keep it natural. When possible, practice and play on natural surfaces, as opposed to artificial turf, which is associated with a high rate of knee injury.

Preventive bracing. If you've had a knee injury before, and you're a down lineman and therefore likely to get hit, you may want to consider being fitted for a preventive brace. No brace is ever going to be able to protect you completely, but it may help to stabilize and support the leg during impact.

BUILD YOUR STRENGTH, FLEXIBILITY, BALANCE, AGILITY, TIMING

R$_x$ *Stretching Workout, ACL Health Workout, General Knee Health Workout*

Golf

Golf isn't high impact, but that doesn't mean there aren't knee problems associated with this sport. The twisting involved with a golf swing puts a lot of strain across the knee joint.

Common injuries: meniscal tear, patellofemoral pain, and injury

HOW TO PROTECT YOURSELF
Use the proper equipment

Clubs. The use of more flexible graphite golf club shafts can reduce the amount of load on the knees, because you don't have to swing as hard.

Use proper footwear. Spikeless shoes allow greater mobility in the foot and leg. Since most courses in the country won't let you anywhere near them in spikes, this won't be an issue for many of you. But if you've been using spikes to hit balls in the backyard, change your shoes.

Train properly

Change your technique. If you're experiencing knee problems, you may want to experiment with alterations to your swing that allow your foot to shift or move instead of staying planted on the ground (which increases torque across the knee). It might hurt your swing, but it'll save your knees.

BUILD YOUR STRENGTH, FLEXIBILITY, BALANCE, AGILITY, TIMING

R$_x$ *Stretching Workout, ACL Health Workout, General Knee Health Workout*

Gymnastics

Gymnastics involves lots of running, jumping, and twisting—all things that put your knee in the line of fire. Proper form often requires hyper-extension when dismounting or tumbling, which means that the leg is fully extended when you land—a recipe for disaster. What's more, gymnastics tends to be a young person's sport, which means that the growth plates, the growing tissue at the end of the bones, are still open, increasing risk of injury.

Common injuries: Osgood-Schlatter's disease, patellar tendinitis, ACL, stress fractures.

HOW TO PROTECT YOURSELF
Train properly

Jump *right*: Many gymnastic maneuvers, done properly, run counter to everything you'd learn in a jumping clinic. But what you do in competition and what you do when you're training don't have to be the same thing. Learn to jump (and to land) properly in practice by bending your knees when you land, engaging the hamstrings, taking the weight off the toes and pushing it back to the heels, and moving as soon as you hit the ground to decrease the forces of deceleration. Then, when you have to stick a landing in competition, you're still staying one step ahead of injury because you've strengthened your decelerators in your training.

BUILD YOUR STRENGTH, FLEXIBILITY, BALANCE, AGILITY, TIMING

R$_x$ *ACL Health Workout, General Knee Health Workout*

Hockey

Hockey players are susceptible to the same kinds of injuries that soccer, rugby, basketball, and football players are, but ACL injuries are less common—there's less friction on the ice. Interestingly, I've noticed that hockey players recover faster from ACL injuries than players from other sports. Since their sense of balance is so exquisitely developed from spending their life on skates, they're more easily able to recruit the nerve receptors they need for stability from other parts of the leg to compensate for the ones they've damaged in the injury.

Common injuries: MCL injury, meniscus tears, ACL injuries

HOW TO PROTECT YOURSELF
Train properly

Agility and balance are essential tools in training your body to protect itself from injury. Keep your knees bent at all times, especially when you cut.

Warm up: Don't think you can get warmed up during play. Skate around the rink at least ten times to get your muscles warm, followed by six forward sprints at half speed so your body gets used to sprinting, and six back sprints at half speed to warm up muscles at the back of the body. Then do my stretching workout, and you'll be ready to play.

BUILD YOUR STRENGTH, FLEXIBILITY, BALANCE, AGILITY, TIMING

Rx | *Stretching Workout, ACL Health Workout, General Knee Health Workout*

Rollerblading

Rollerblading involves a lot of lateral leg movement, which can result in a lot of overuse problems if you're not careful. As in skiing, you're attaching extenders to the foot, so the knee is especially at risk.

Common injuries: IT band syndrome, patellofemoral pain

How to Protect Yourself
Use the proper equipment

Wear knee pads. Knee pads should be adequately padded and fit well.

Buy blades that fit. Make sure the heel doesn't move up and down in the boot.

Build Your Strength, Flexibility, Balance, Agility, Timing

R$_x$ *Stretching Workout, General Knee Health Workout*

Because Rollerblading involves so much lateral movement, it's especially important to make sure that there's balance between the inner and outer muscles in the leg.

Running

The American Academy of Orthopedic Surgeons estimates that one out of every five runners gets a knee injury over the course of a year. A great many of my patients are runners—and a great number of their injuries could have been prevented.

Common injuries. "Runner's knee" (patellofemoral disorders), iliotibial band syndrome, tendinitis; pes anserine bursitis, stress fractures

How to Protect Yourself
Use the proper equipment

Use proper footwear. Buy good shoes. That doesn't necessarily mean the most expensive pair, just the best ones for your feet. You'll find guidelines for selecting the right footwear on pages 70-71—this information is especially important for runners. Run in the shoe before you buy it! Walking around doesn't tell you how a shoe will fit when you're running, and running in place isn't quite the same thing either.

Replace your shoes often. Just because the tops of your shoes still look brand-new doesn't mean they are. The ability of a running shoe to absorb shock decreases pretty rapidly, especially when you're logging many miles. If you're running 20 miles a week, you'll need new shoes every four to six months. As a general rule of thumb, you should replace your shoes every 250 to 400 miles. If you run often (over 30 miles a week), change them at 250; if you run less (under 30 a week), it's OK to wait a little longer.

Train properly

Don't do too much too soon. The likelihood of an overuse injury increases when you try to do too much too soon. If you're just getting back into condition, do a little less than you think you can to begin. Gradually ease yourself into sprints and speed work and hills— downhill running especially exacerbates patellofemoral pain. Your training should include easy weeks as well as easy days.

Rest. Runners who run more than 40 miles a week have higher injury rates, and those who run seven days a week without rest days are injured more as well.

Run on the right surface. The surface you're running on should have some give, especially when returning to running from an injury. Look for free-floating platforms on treadmills, where the platform is independent from the machine and has its own shocks (these are standard at most high-end gyms). If you're running outside, asphalt is better than concrete, and a smooth dirt road is even better than asphalt. Change direction often on crowned surfaces, like a banked road, and don't run too often in the same direction on a track; the uneven loads on the knees can cause overuse injuries. Avoid running downhill for long periods of time.

Use proper technique. If you have chronic and consistent knee pain, it might be the result of poor gait habits. It's worth it to be assessed by a professional. A gait coach will actually run behind you, analyze your stride, and train you to correct bad habits. (You can find a gait coach through your local runners' club.)

BUILD YOUR STRENGTH, FLEXIBILITY, BALANCE, AGILITY, TIMING

R$_X$ | *Stretching Workout, General Knee Health Workout*

Regular stretching may help reduce injuries. Because so much of a runner's emphasis is on acceleration, which requires the muscles at the front of the leg, runners frequently develop tightness in the posterior muscle groups, including the hamstrings, calf muscles, and lateral groups, most specifically the iliotibial band. And don't forget about your core strength, as so many runners do!

Skiing

Knee injuries account for well over a quarter of all downhill ski injuries, making them the most common injuries seen in downhill skiers. When you ski, you're locked into big extenders on your feet; these transfer forces across the knee, especially if they get caught and don't release. Although MCL sprains are the most frequent knee injury, the ACL is injured in approximately 20 percent of all ski injuries.

Common Injuries: MCL, ACL, meniscal tears, fractures

HOW TO PROTECT YOURSELF
Use the proper equipment

Update and maintain your equipment. Use current equipment—it's safer. Have your bindings serviced by a ski mechanic every 15 to 30 ski days, or at least at the start of the ski season. There's a high correlation between how frequently downhill skiers have their bindings tested and the incidence of lower-leg injuries. Test the release mechanism on your boots yourself every time you put them on. Make sure your boots fit, so you won't loosen the buckles for comfort, and decrease your ability to control your skis. Make sure your bindings aren't too tight. The American Society for Testing and Materials has defined standard release settings for alpine ski bindings, based on the age, body weight, and type of skier using them. Those standards should be followed by the person adjusting your bindings.

Consider preventive bracing. If you've already had an injury, use very good protective braces. The use of prophylactic or functional knee braces to decrease the risk of knee ligament injuries is controversial. Pull-on neoprene-like knee sleeves are fine for mild support and comfort and they can be helpful with meniscal symptoms or patellofemoral pain.

Train Properly

Take lessons. The better trained the skier, the less likely injury will occur. Lessons are especially important if you're just starting the sport, but even veterans should think about a refresher course. Training techniques have changed considerably since your dad learned to ski, and the sport has also gotten safer as a result.

Slow down. Speed is dangerous, the same way it is in a car—the faster you're going, the more serious the injury will be.

Avoid high-risk behavior. Slowing down is just the first step. Avoid high-risk behavior in general, like skiing too fast on an overcrowded slope, skiing in an off-limit area, on a poorly groomed slope, or on one above your capability level. Follow the rules of the slope.

Learn how to fall. That means falling, not trying to stop the fall. It also means falling forward. Try not to hyperextend your knees. Don't try to get up if you're still sliding down the hill, and don't try to get up from an awkward position on the ground.

Beware of the chair lift! One skier stepping on the back of another's skis as they're getting off the chairlift is a leading cause of ski injuries. Sit on the outside, and avoid snowboarders if you can; the way they get off the lift increases the likelihood that they'll trap one of your skis.

BUILD YOUR STRENGTH, FLEXIBILITY, BALANCE, AGILITY, TIMING

R$_X$ *ACL Health Workout, Stretching Workout*

Sometimes we can get out on the slopes only a couple of times a year, but it's important to train for those few days year-round.

Soccer

Soccer, like basketball, is a sport that requires lots of quick cuts, pivots, sudden stops, and turns. The knee bears up to seven times your body weight when you kick the ball. Knee injuries count for 16 to 25 percent of all soccer injuries.

Common injuries: MCL, meniscus tear, ACL, patellofemoral pain, patellar/quad tendinitis

HOW TO PROTECT YOURSELF
Use the proper equipment

Footwear. Use molded cleats or ribbed soles. Screw-in cleats are associated with a higher rate of injury, but can be used if conditions are appropriate (i.e., on wet, muddy fields).

Keep it natural: When possible, practice and play on natural surfaces, as opposed to artificial turf, which is associated with a high rate of knee injury.

BUILD YOUR STRENGTH, FLEXIBILITY, BALANCE, AGILITY, TIMING

R_x *The General Knee Health Workout, ACL Health Workout, Stretching Workout*

Strength Training

It's not a cutting sport, like football or hockey, but a surprising number of knee injuries arise as a result of weight lifting and strength training.

Common injuries: patellar tendinitis, patellofemoral pain, meniscus tears

HOW TO PROTECT YOURSELF
Train properly

Use the whole leg. Perform each exercise through a (pain-free) maximum range of motion.

Train the back as well as the front. We have a tendency to focus on the body parts we see in the mirror. Don't neglect the back of the body as well.

Give your muscles enough time to recover. Work alternate muscle groups every day. **Always work the large muscles *first*.**

BUILD YOUR STRENGTH, FLEXIBILITY, BALANCE, AGILITY, TIMING

R_x *General Knee Health Workout, Stretching Workout*

Swimming

Swimming is generally low impact, but the use of the breaststroke whip kick can result in overuse injuries.

Common injuries: breaststroker's knee (patellofemoral pain), MCL sprain, plica injury

BUILD YOUR STRENGTH, FLEXIBILITY, BALANCE, AGILITY, TIMING

R_x *General Knee Health Workout, Stretching Workout*

Tennis

Like all sports that require you to run and change direction rapidly, tennis can result in knee pain and injury.

Common injuries: patellofemoral pain, ACL injury, meniscal tears

HOW TO PROTECT YOURSELF
Use the proper equipment

Get proper footwear. It's essential to buy shoes designed specifically for tennis to ensure that you have the kind of support your knee requires.

Surface. If possible, avoid playing on surfaces with no "give." Every step you take on a cement, asphalt, or synthetic court sends shock waves up the leg and through the knee. If you play on these surfaces, make sure your footwear is adequately cushioned, and consider wearing cushioning inserts in your shoes as a supplement. These surfaces also grab your shoes more firmly than clay or grass, which means that it's more likely that your foot will stay put while your leg moves, causing a twisting injury.

BUILD YOUR STRENGTH, FLEXIBILITY, BALANCE, AGILITY, TIMING

R_x *General Knee Health Workout; ACL Injury Prevention Workout; Stretching Workout*

Volleyball

Common injuries: Jumper's knee, ACL injury, bone contusion, Osgood-Schlatter's disease, iliotibial band syndrome.

HOW TO PROTECT YOURSELF
Use the proper equipment

Use knee pads. Wear knee pads to protect yourself when you're diving for a ball and end up on the court.

Look at your playing surface. When possible, practice and play on wooden or synthetic elastic surfaces. Harder floors, such as concrete, put too much stress on the leg.

Train properly

Jump right. With a little training, you can learn to jump right—in a way that jeopardizes your knee the least. Keep your knees aligned and underneath you at all times, instead of allowing them to splay out. As you land, use your hamstrings, not just your quads, and shift your weight from your toes to your mid-foot, like a rocking chair, and keep your knees bent. Keep moving after landing, so your body doesn't have to decelerate quite as much.

Call the ball. Communicate with the other players on the court so you're less likely to get into a collision with one of your teammates.

Yoga

The stretching aspect of yoga is terrific, but certain poses, especially if incorrectly taught, can wreak havoc on the knees.

Common injuries: patellofemoral problems, meniscus tears

HOW TO PROTECT YOURSELF
Train properly

Listen to your body, especially if it's telling you something different than the instructor is. Use pain as a guide. If something hurts, you're either doing it wrong, or it's something that's not good for you. In either case, you shouldn't be doing it. Some poses to avoid if you have knee problems:

Hero (*Virasana*): This is the pose where you kneel, with your rear end on the ground between your knees. It causes a tremendous amount of torque on the knee, and should be avoided if you have existing knee problems.

Lotus (*Padmasana*): A cross-legged pose that involves putting both feet on the thighs, which is a very deep stretch for the outside of the legs and can stress the knees.

Warrior (*Virabhadrasana*): In this pose, the front leg is deeply bent, and the back leg is planted at an angle and completely straight. This can cause an inordinate amount of strain on both knees.

> **Note**: In all bent-knee poses, remember that the knee should never be farther ahead than the foot.

BUILD YOUR STRENGTH, FLEXIBILITY, BALANCE, AGILITY, TIMING

R_X *General Knee Health Workout*

While yoga is a great all-round exercise, and certainly works to increase flexibility, it shouldn't be viewed as a substitute for rehabilitation after an injury, since it doesn't isolate all the muscles as well as a strength-training workout.

The safer you play and train, the longer you'll be able to do it comfortably and without injury. It's worth taking necessary precautions and investing in the right equipment.

PART III

KNEE PAIN AND INJURY

■ CHAPTER EIGHT ■

FINDING A DOCTOR

So you've injured yourself, or you've been experiencing chronic knee pain and none of the do-it-yourself remedies has worked to permanently alleviate the pain. It's time for a trip to the doctor. How will you go about finding one?

The first step is to ask a doctor with whom you already have a trusting professional relationship for a recommendation. He or she is going to refer you to someone good because it reflects well on them, and more important, your doctor wants to facilitate the best care possible for you. So if you have a good relationship with your general practitioner, ask their office to refer you to a good specialist.

Most of my patients end up in my office through word of mouth—they found me through another one of my patients. If I'm looking for a specialist for my kids or myself, I ask around to see if anyone in my circle has a doctor they like.

If you're not having any luck through word of mouth, you can always contact one of the two organizations below. Both have websites that feature "find a member doctor" services, searchable by area. The American Medical Society for Sports Medicine (AMSSM) members are predominantly nonoperating sports medicine doctors; The American Orthopaedic Society for Sports Medicine (AOSSM) members are predominantly surgeons.

> The American Medical Society for Sports Medicine (AMSSM)
> 11639 Earnshaw
> Overland Park, KS 66210
> Phone: 913-327-1415
> Fax: 913-327-1491
> *www.amssm.org*

> The American Orthopaedic Society for Sports Medicine (AOSSM)
> 6300 North River Road, Suite 500
> Rosemont, IL 60018
> Toll-free phone: 877-321-3500
> Phone: 847-292-4900
> Fax: 847-292-4905
> *www.sportsmed.org*

What to Look For in a Doctor

Obviously, you're looking for a physician licensed to practice in your state. If there's any question as to whether your doctor is licensed and in good standing, you can contact:

> Federation of State Medical Boards of the United States, Inc.
> PO Box 619850
> Dallas, TX 75261-9850
> Phone: 817- 868-4000
> Fax: 817- 868-4099
> *www.fsmb.org*

Your doctor should also be *board-certified*, which means that he or she has gone through a special training process and has passed national board exams, which gives them specialty certification by one of the twenty-four member boards of the American Board of Medical Specialties (ABMS). You can confirm certification by contacting:

The American Board of Medical Specialties
Phone: 866-ASK-ABMS (275-2267)
or use the "Who's Certified" link: ***www.abms.org***

Your doctor should be affiliated with a hospital of good reputation. The magazine *US News & World Report* publishes an annual ranking of the best hospitals in the country, divided by specialty. You can find orthopedic rankings under "Best Hospitals" on their website: ***www.usnews.com.***

An academic appointment certainly isn't necessary, but it generally means that the doctor is up to date on the emerging technologies and procedures in the field. You may also want to inquire if the doctor has published anything recently: an academic publication, especially an article that deals specifically with your condition, is a good indication that someone is really interested in a particular problem and is not only up to date but participating in the emerging research.

Those are the basics. But finding the *right* doctor for you requires that you do a little more homework.

Like all professionals, doctors approach what they do with a certain perspective, one that's formed by their training, background, experience, personal philosophies about medicine, and their personalities. How will you discover how your physician thinks?

More and more doctors have websites, and you can find out a great deal about a doctor, including their educational background and their specialties from them. If your doctor doesn't have a website, or there's additional information you need, feel free to call the office and talk to a member of the staff. Some questions you might want to ask include: Does the doctor specialize in a specific body part (the knee, shoulder, or hip, for instance)? Does he have a lot of experience with my particular injury? If you're looking for a surgeon, it's appropriate to ask how many of these procedures she's done in the last year, and what hospitals she's affiliated with. One important question to ask the doctor or staff is whether or not it's OK to call with questions, and how quickly they'll respond. If you'd like more information, you can ask for a phone consultation with the doctor. I have noticed some shared characteristics among the really good physicians I know, and I think it's worth sharing them here.

They listen to the patient. One of my professors once said that you can diagnose almost any injury just by listening to the patient: "the patient will tell you what's wrong with him." Listening to a patient encourages him to participate in his own treatment and recovery, and it's also the most efficient way to come to a diagnosis. How the injury occurred, what noise or sensation you heard as it was happening, and what you felt immediately afterward can give a good doctor as many clues as the physical exam does.

They treat the whole patient. If you have knee pain or a knee injury, you know that there are a number of factors that go into every treatment decision. Before one treatment option over another is recommended for a patient, a host of issues must be taken into account. Some involve the knee: How bad is the injury? How long has it been like this? Is it showing signs of improvement? Does it interfere with your ability to get around and live your life?

But many of the questions have nothing to do with the joint itself. Questions like: How old are you? How active are you? Could you commit to losing fifteen pounds? What's your occupation? Do you need your knee in your work? Would you be able to take three or four weeks off work while you recuperated from surgery? Would your employer allow you to work from home? Would you be able to carry out a program of physical therapy? If your insurance doesn't cover all of the expense, would you comfortably be able to make up the difference? The answer to these questions guide treatment recommendations as well.

They treat the patient, not just the injury. It's also part of the physician's job to help their patients integrate their diagnosis into their lives. If the ultimate goal was simply to keep knees safe, we'd tell everybody to stop skiing, stop playing basketball, and stop running around after their kids. But that's no life! The ultimate goal is to manage pain and injury effectively, so that people who have knee problems can stay active and enjoy their lives. To do that, the doctor and the patient have to become partners in order to figure out how best to integrate the knee problem into the patient's life.

Let's say you're an electrician, someone in good shape, and you've torn your ACL. Given your profession, the injury, and your physical condition, surgery is probably the best treatment option for you. But, for reasons of your own, you're adamant about not wanting to go through with a reconstruction. Your doctor has a responsibility to tell you why he or she feels that surgery is their preference for you, and once you have that information you can make an informed decision. If the result of that informed decision means that you don't pursue surgery, then the next step is for you and your doctor to come up with a way to manage your risk.

After the diagnosis, your doctor needs to ask some more questions: What are you willing to give up? What's non-negotiable? Would you settle for two sets of tennis instead of three? Ideally, you'll end up with a compromise that's specific to your case—your injury and the activities you want to participate in. These negotiations may not be guaranteed to keep knees 100 percent safe, but they provide a more realistic approach than just telling an active person to discontinue activity altogether. It also teaches the patient to begin to factor risk into the choices they make—and that means fewer re-injuries in the long run.

The Second Opinion

If for any reason you feel shaky about the diagnosis or the treatment recommendations you've received, you have every right to pursue a second opinion. In fact, some insurance companies require that you get one before surgery. Certainly you shouldn't hesitate if you think you'd like to see another doctor. Your doctor may even recommend that you get one if you're not getting better as fast as he'd like to you to, or because he wants confirmation of a diagnosis, or just the added comfort of another set of eyes. I see plenty of patients for my colleagues; if a second opinion is what it takes to give a patient the best care possible, there's no reason not to pursue that option.

Your Relationship with Your Doctor

Establishing a positive doctor-patient relationship is an investment in your care. The relationship you have with your doctor may matter a lot or only a little, depending on your personality. The most important thing is that you trust that you're getting the best care possible.

For instance, a friend of mine goes to a neurologist who has the worst bedside manner of all time. He can barely be bothered to grunt hello when she walks in the door, but she doesn't care. Her condition had declined under a number of doctors with much better personalities, and she believes, with some good reason, that the somewhat unconventional therapy he recommended for her saved her life. She'd follow him to the ends of the earth, even if he can't be bothered to say hello.

Other people do need more of a personal relationship. A woman recently came to see me for a second opinion about a meniscal tear. She wasn't unhappy or unsure about the diagnosis and treatment path the first doctor had given her—she just hadn't liked him because he was too "jocky." I personally think it's a silly reason to leave a good doctor, but I respect her right to feel comfortable with her physician.

Some patients want to participate in decisions about their care—and some don't. One of my own patients, a high-powered executive, didn't want to know anything about his treatment—he wanted me to "take care of it." In other words, he wanted to delegate his knee the same way he delegated marketing and sales chores in his company. But that's not the way this works. Sure, I could "fix" his knee by making his treatment decisions for him, but it would just be a waste of time if he wasn't willing to take some ownership of his knee and its rehabilitation, and that's something you can't outsource. He had to be dragged kicking and screaming to the understanding that unless he was willing to act as a full participant in his recuperation, he'd be very unhappy with the outcome.

I tell these stories for one reason: only you know what you need from your relationship with a doctor. You have a right to feel comfortable, listened to, and most important, to feel that you're receiving the absolute best care possible.

CHAPTER NINE

ARRIVING AT A DIAGNOSIS

Your injury has brought you to a doctor's office. How will she arrive at a diagnosis? Total patient care means more than just looking at a knee under a bell jar. There's no fancy technological substitute for a doctor putting her hands on a patient's leg and actually feeling what's going on inside it. So I'd like to encourage you to give equal weight to all the aspects of the process that lead to your doctor's diagnosis.

Patient History

One of the most revealing pieces of information you can give your doctor is an accurate history of how your knee pain developed, so be prepared to describe exactly how the pain started. Here are some of the questions you may be asked:

— Have you had a knee problem before?

— Is the pain you're experiencing now the result of an injury?

— If yes, was your leg hit, did you hit something—in other words, was it a contact injury?

— Were you able to continue what you were doing when you got injured, or were you forced to stop immediately?

— Did you hear a noise when it happened, like a pop?

— How soon after the injury did your knee swell (within the first 24 hours)?

— Has the swelling subsided and come back since the injury?

— Is the pain dull? sharp?

— Where in the knee does it hurt?

— Is the pain on the inside of the knee, or the outside? Is it under the kneecap, or deep inside the knee?

— Is it worse when you go up or down stairs?

— Can you lunge? twist? kneel?

— Does it hurt after you've been sitting for a long time?

— Does it hurt or is it stiff first thing in the morning, before you've worked it out a little?

— Does it lock on you so you can't straighten it fully, or bend it past a certain degree? Does it give out as if you're going to fall?

— Does the pain wake you at night?

Your responses to these questions are an important factor in the ultimate diagnosis of your injury. Next, a general medical history is taken. Your doctor will ask you about any existing medical problems, like diabetes, high blood pressure, allergies, previous surgeries, and whether you're on any medication. She'll probably ask you what kind of work you do, if you exercise and what type and how often, and whether or not you smoke. These medical and lifestyle details will be pertinent in going forward with treatment.

Diagnostic Tests

An experienced doctor can diagnose almost any knee problem, simply by noticing the way a patient's leg reacts when it's bearing weight and when it's physically manipulated.

So one of the first things your doctor will do is watch the way you walk into a room—whether you limp or not and how you're protecting your leg. She'll also check your alignment: whether you're flat-footed or not, which way your shinbones rotate, whether you're bow-legged or knock-kneed—all the issues that we've discussed that contribute to knee pain.

Establishing a Baseline

Your doctor will test both your injured and your uninjured side in order to establish a "baseline." Some people naturally have more play than others in the structures of the joints, and it's important to establish what's normal for your knees by checking the response of the uninvolved leg first.

The next step is for your doctor to touch or palpate your leg, looking for signs of swelling or tenderness. She'll evaluate your range of motion in both the knee and the hip, which may be referring pain to the knee. The amount of flexibility you have in your hamstrings and quads can also alert her to a possible problem; many of the most common knee injuries result at least partially from tight muscles, especially in the back of the body.

She'll also look to see if there's been any atrophy—wasting or weakening—in the muscles in the thigh, particularly the quads, and she may test the timing of the muscles in the thigh to see if a stronger outside muscle is firing before a weaker inner one, putting uneven stresses on the kneecap itself.

She will test your kneecap, to see how it's moving within the trochlear groove. She'll push it into the femur (a move known as the patellofemoral grind test) to see if there is noise or pain. She may also try to get it to "jump the track" to see if the structures holding it in place are intact.

She will straighten and extend the leg and listen closely for any crunching, or *crepitus*, as the leg moves.

The next level is a series of tests that puts specific stresses on the knee in order to determine the knee's stability.

One of the best indicators of anterior cruciate ligament (ACL) stability is the **Lachman test**. Your doctor will hold your thigh still and pull your lower leg forward with your knee bent (to 20–30 degrees of flexion) in order to see if the knee is loose. If there is "increased translation"— in other words, if the lower leg moves farther forward than normal—then your ACL may have been compromised. Your doctor will always compare the involved knee to the normal one.

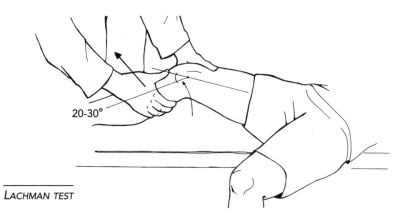

20-30°

LACHMAN TEST

In the **pivot shift test** your doctor holds your leg under her arm while she applies force to the outside of your leg and internally rotates your shinbone in order to see if the shinbone moves while you're bending or straightening your leg. If you've torn your ACL, it actually feels as if the shinbone jumps over the thighbone, sometimes accompanied by a clunking noise.

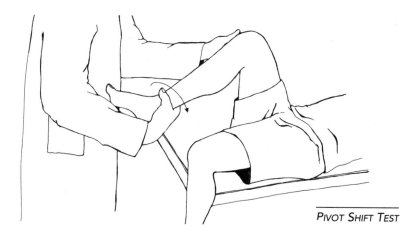

PIVOT SHIFT TEST

The **anterior drawer test** is another, less sensitive way of determining if the ACL has been damaged. You lie on your back, with your knee bent and the foot of the injured leg flat on the table, as if standing. Your doctor will grasp the top of your calf and attempt to pull your lower leg forward, toward herself. If there's increased translation, something may be wrong.

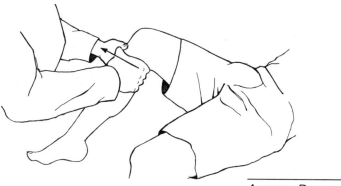

ANTERIOR DRAWER TEST

The **posterior drawer test** is essentially the same test done in reverse, in order to determine if there's a problem with the posterior cruciate ligament (PCL). Your doctor pushes your bent leg back toward your body, to determine whether a damaged ligament is allowing the leg to move farther back than normal. Your doctor may also simply look at your legs while your feet are on the table or raised in the air so that your shins are parallel to the table—if your lower leg appears to be sagging backward on the involved side, it's a sign that the PCL may be compromised.

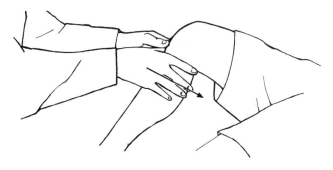

POSTERIOR DRAWER TEST

To see if your MCL is damaged, your doctor will hold your slightly bent (30 to 45 degrees) leg and apply pressure to the outside of the knee. If your lower leg can move outward more than normal, then you may have a tear in the liga-ment; this test is called a **valgus stress test**. The

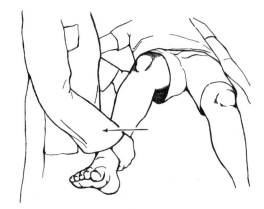

VALGUS STRESS TEST

same test in reverse, called a **varus stress test**, is done to check the LCL.

In **McMurray's test**, you lie on your back while your doctor puts a stress on the knee while turning your ankle so that your shinbone is rotating outward and inward. The leg is bent past 90 degrees and straightened. This twists and compresses the meniscus, and the presence of pain, resistance, or a clunking sound will alert your doctor to a tear.

During the **Apley test**, you're lying on your stomach with your knee flexed and the foot at a 90 degree angle to your body. If the meniscus is damaged, you will feel pain when your doctor applies downward pressure to your foot with one arm while twisting the lower leg with his hands.

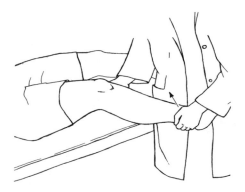

VARUS STRESS TEST

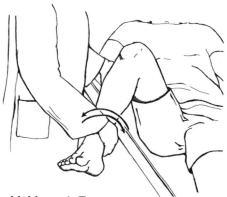

MCMURRAY'S TEST

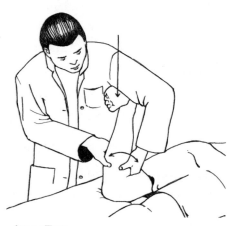

APLEY TEST

Imaging Technology

By the time the physical examination is complete, your doctor will probably have a pretty good idea of what's wrong with your knee. The next step is to confirm the diagnosis—and make sure that other parts of the knee haven't been damaged as well—by ordering more sophisticated tests that use technology to photograph the knee's inner structures.

X Ray

X rays are a form of energy that passes through tissues and makes a picture—like a shadow—onto film. They're mostly useful to tell us if anything's wrong with your bones. They'll show a fracture, bone spurs, and osteoarthritis, alignment issues, as well as abnormalities of the growth plates, and they'll tell us if a piece of bone has broken off with a torn tendon; however, they won't directly alert us to anything wrong with the soft structures in the knee.

Magnetic Resonance Imagery (MRI)

When you get an MRI, you usually lie inside a huge tube that makes a lot of noise, and "pictures" are taken of your tissues using magnetic waves moving around the tube. The level of detail an MRI affords your doctor is truly astonishing, especially because you can see a much greater range of tissues—including the menisci, ligaments, tendons, and muscles in and about the knee.

It's not for the claustrophobic (or for anyone with any metal in their bodies, like a pacemaker), but this test can really help your doctor to isolate the injury or injuries causing your pain.

Ultrasound

Ultrasound uses sound waves to make a picture. A gel is applied to the skin, and a probe is moved over the affected area. This is the same technology used to do sonograms during pregnancy. It's quicker and less expensive than an MRI, and it's usually used in the knee to assess tendinitis in the patella, quadriceps, or hamstring, or to see if there's a popliteal cyst in the back of the knee. I prefer the MRI because it shows us all this and more, but it does cost more.

KT1000/2000

The KT1000 is basically a drawer test, like the anterior and posterior drawer test your doctor will have performed during your physical exam. The difference is simply that an instrument does the pulling and measures the amount of laxity—the amount that the lower leg can move in relation to the upper leg. This helps to assess the degree of instability in the knee, and therefore the grade of the sprain in a ligament. The KT2000 is a slightly newer and more advanced instrument.

Blood Tests

If your knee is badly swollen, with no apparent injury or cause, we'll give you a blood test, which can help to rule out a variety of conditions including rheumatoid arthritis, lupus, Lyme disease, and gout.

Aspiration

At times, doctors will aspirate the knee, which means that they insert a needle into the joint itself and remove some of the fluid inside.

Called "tapping the knee," this can

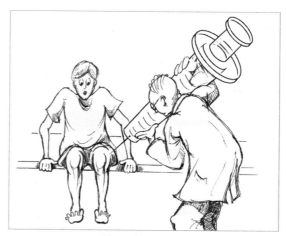

KNEE ASPIRATION

act as both a diagnosis and a treatment. If the knee is badly swollen, a great deal of relief is to be had by removing some of the fluid inside. The state of the fluid can also provide us with diagnostic clues. Blood indicates that some part of the knee, like a torn ACL, is bleeding into the joint. If the liquid is filled with crystals, you may have gout. Fat globules suggest a fracture; cloudy fluid may be sign of an infection.

Arthroscopy

Arthroscopy is a surgical technique that can also be used to clarify a diagnosis, but is mostly used to address a definitive problem. The word is derived from the Greek: *arthro* means "joint," and the verb *skopein* means "to look," so arthroscopy means to look inside the joint. And that's literally what it means. During arthroscopy, your surgeon will insert a tiny light and lens system into a small incision in your leg. This system will illuminate and magnify the inside of your knee. More than one incision may be necessary to get a full view of the interior.

In most cases, if the surgeon discovers a torn meniscus or similar injury in the course of the arthroscopy, he will fix it while he's in there.

In the past, arthroscopy was recommended as a diagnostic tool whenever there was bleeding in the joint, but most injuries, including ACL injuries, can be diagnosed accurately in 95 percent of cases with a full medical history (including detail about the injury) and physical exam, using an MRI and other technologies when necessary.

CHAPTER TEN

THE MOST COMMON KNEE PROBLEMS

I n the following sections, we'll be looking at some of the most common knee problems and how they happen, how you can recognize their symptoms, how your doctor will diagnose them, and what your treatment options are.

It is my intention to empower you to make intelligent decisions about your knee health, but I want to remind you that no book can ever replace a relationship with a doctor familiar with your medical history, physical condition, and individual injury. I can make generalizations about the relative merits and disadvantages of surgery for a certain population, but ultimately, it's a decision that has to be made by you and your doctor. My comments are intended to serve as a springboard for discussions with your doctor; please treat them as such.

If you take one concept away from this chapter, I hope it's that *the individualization of the treatment plan is as important as an accurate diagnosis*. This is how I define total patient care.

Treatment decisions are *always* multifactored. For instance, some of my patients, as long as they can get around and don't have any associated injuries, choose to go without surgery for an injury like a torn ACL. This is a decision that we have made together, based on their function and personal goals. Another concept that I'd like you to take away is the idea of educating yourself so that you can manage your own risk. A colleague of mine, a sports medicine doctor, has been walking around on two completely torn ACLs for ten years. He doesn't want surgery— his knees don't bother him, and he doesn't want to take the time or deal with the problems associated with surgery. He knows the risks, and he's managing them. He's in terrific condition, and makes sure he has strong dynamic stabilizers to compensate for the lost ligaments. But he's picked and chosen the activities he will participate in, based on their risk. He doesn't play basketball once a week anymore, or competitive tennis games, but since he loves to ski, and only gets to do it one week a year, he puts on his braces and takes the risk.

Recovery—and your expectations for your own recovery—must also be personalized. Many factors influence how fast you recover from an injury. Some, like your age and genes, are out of your control; others, like how much energy you put into your rehab, are not. At the end of the day, all these factors, combined with the severity of the injury and whether other parts of the knee were injured, determine how fast you'll recover. I hope you'll consider the following recovery parameters as guidelines, not hard and fast rules. You'll get the best results if you pay attention to your body's needs, and show patience with it as it heals at its own pace.

The Ligaments

As you'll remember, there are four major ligaments in the knee. These act as restraints on the joint, controlling the range of motion permitted to the leg.

When something forces the knee past the range of motion permitted by the ligament, the ligament may stretch and eventually tear. Since the ligaments are made of many tightly woven strands, a tear may range from minor to complete.

Ligament injuries are graded by severity: a Grade I, or simple, sprain is a microtear or extreme stretch; the ligament may be painful but is fundamentally stable. A Grade II sprain is a more serious tear, and the ligament is less stable; and a Grade III sprain is a complete tear. These are considered severe sprains. Since Grade III sprains may damage the nerves in and around the ligament, there may be less pain associated with these more severe injuries. Since ligament sprains tend to cause pain and swelling, your doctor may ask you to rest and ice the injury for a few days before confirming the diagnosis.

The four ligaments fall into two categories: the cruciate ligaments, which are located inside the joint itself, and the collateral ligaments, which run along the inner and outer sides of the leg.

The Cruciate Ligaments

The two cruciate ligaments, the anterior cruciate (ACL) at the front and the posterior cruciate (PCL) at the back, are located inside the knee joint itself, connecting the thighbone to the shin. They cross, making an X inside the joint, which explains their name: the word "cruciate" means "cross."

The cruciate ligaments suffer damage when the lower leg is forced too far forward, backward, or is rotated too much.

ANTERIOR CRUCIATE LIGAMENT (ACL)

The anterior cruciate ligament, located inside the joint and at the front, exists to prevent the lower leg from moving too far forward. When something forces the lower leg farther forward than the ACL can comfortably allow, this ligament can stretch or tear, partially or completely. The ACL also tightens when the knee is twisted or extended, thus when the shin is rotated too much from the thigh, or over-straightened too suddenly, the ACL can suffer injury.

ACL injuries are the most common ligament injuries, and they are a particular problem for female athletes.

HOW CAN I INJURE MY ACL?

ACL injuries are often found in sports such as football, basketball, and skiing, which require twisting motions through the leg while the foot stays planted on the ground. You can injure your ACL by suddenly changing direction while you're running, decelerating rapidly, by turning quickly without lifting your foot, by landing incorrectly from a jump. Direct contact is also a culprit.

HOW WILL I KNOW IF I'VE INJURED MY ACL?

Symptoms differ, but most people describe hearing a pop in their leg, or the feeling that something has snapped—this is the sound of the ligament itself, snapping like a rubber band. The knee usually swells fairly rapidly (within two hours after the injury), because the torn ligament is bleeding into the joint. This is called a *hemeoarthrosis*. The most common complaint is pain; the feeling that the leg is giving out completely, or buckling when weight is put on it is a close second.

HOW WILL MY DOCTOR DIAGNOSE AN ACL INJURY?

Your doctor will take a history of the injury and then do a physical exam to determine whether or not the ACL has been damaged. The physical will include the Lachman test and the pivot shift test.

Your doctor may also use MRIs and X rays to confirm the diagnosis and determine whether there has been any associated damage to the cartilage and bone in the knee. Instrument devices like a KT1000 are often used to document the increased movement of the shin and the thighbone, which helps assess the degree of instability and can help diagnose the grade of the sprain.

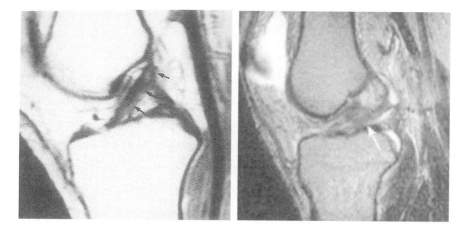

MRI OF NORMAL ACL   MRI OF TORN ACL

WHAT ARE MY TREATMENT OPTIONS?

There are both surgical and nonsurgical treatment options available to treat an ACL injury. Your doctor's recommendation will be based on a number of factors, including the acuteness (how recent) and the severity of the injury; the apparent stability of the knee; other injuries to the knee sustained at the same time; your age; your ability to comply with rehabilitation; and your activity level.

You can live with an ACL tear without ever fixing it. Many people do, especially people with low activity levels, no other associated knee injury, and only mild laxity or instability in the leg when it's examined.

People who cannot comply with rehab should also consider taking a more conservative approach. But you shouldn't live with an ACL tear without treating it, through the steps outlined below. If left untreated, whether surgically or through rehabilitation, ACL injuries can cause a great deal of pain and instability in the leg, as well as meniscal tears and a high risk of early osteoarthritis.

NON-SURGICAL TREATMENT OPTIONS

A stretched ACL often does not require surgery, and in some cases even partially torn ACLs will mend nicely with the proper care and rehabilitation.

Remember, choosing to go with non-surgical treatments right now doesn't mean you can't have surgery later. In fact, recent studies have indicated that ACL reconstructions are more successful when the joint has returned to the full range of motion. Even if you end up opting for surgery, you can use these non-surgical treatments in the meantime.

RICE. Rest, ice, compression, and elevation, combined with NSAIDs, can help to alleviate the pain and speed healing. Relative rest is especially important: running or putting too much pressure on an unstable ACL can cause damage to the meniscus, the cartilage in the center of the knee. Crutches are indicated for the first few days, until the pain abates and weight-bearing can be tolerated. While rest is important, ice and compression to quickly decrease the swelling allow earlier full range of motion, which is a priority.

Aspiration. A needle may be inserted into the joint to withdraw some of the fluid and blood causing the swelling. This is most often not needed, but can be done if the swelling is causing excruciating pain, or as a diagnosis to determine if there is blood in the knee joint. (Blood would suggest an ACL tear, but can also be seen in patellar dislocation, peripheral meniscal tears, other ligament injuries, or fractures.)

Bracing. The knee may remain relatively unstable with certain activities, and your doctor may recommend a specially fitted, hinged, de-rotational brace to stabilize the knee and prevent re-injury during activities that put strain on the knee. Sometimes a non-hinged, well-supported knee sleeve with a hole for the kneecap is used right after the injury for compression and mild stabilization. These are available from a pharmacy.

Physical therapy. After a short period of rest, the focus of rehabilitation is to strengthen the muscles around the knee, especially the hamstrings, to compensate for the compromised ligament without putting undue strain on the already damaged joint. Therapy should include exercises like those found in my ACL Health Workout.

SURGICAL OPTIONS

Surgery is recommended for many, from the young (early teens) to the older (late middle age). This applies to the active person, especially if you have other ligament injuries or associated meniscal tears in the injured knee. These are people who are unlikely to respond well to a more conservative approach. Surgery is also indicated when a non-surgical approach has failed to stabilize the knee. A completely torn ACL does not repair itself, and how your body accommodates this will play a role in your decision to have surgery.

Talk to your doctor about the timing of the surgery. In some cases, there are benefits to delaying the procedure for a period of time. Studies have shown, for instance, that you are likely to experience less post-surgical scarring and stiffness from an ACL reconstruction if you wait until you have regained full range of motion before undergoing the procedure.

ACL repair. If the ligament has been torn in the middle, it can be repaired by sewing the ends together, but these direct repairs are unsuccessful. If you choose the surgical route, I would suggest reconstruction instead.

ACL reconstruction. ACL reconstruction is almost always done arthroscopically. In this procedure, the ends of the torn ACL are removed and a strip of tissue is threaded through the joint to connect the thighbone to the shinbone, mimicking the natural function of the ACL.

ACL GRAFT CHOICES

In order to reconstruct your ACL, your surgeon will need to get the material to work with, either from somewhere else in your body or somewhere else entirely. The two primary options are autografts and allografts.

Graft materials that are taken from other places in the patient are called **autografts**. The most common grafts are the patellar tendon, which connects the kneecap to the shin, and the hamstring tendon. Because the hamstrings themselves are so strong, removing these tendons doesn't do much to affect the stability of the leg.

It is difficult to demonstrate surgical outcome differences between a patellar tendon and a hamstring tendon graft. The hamstring is generally less painful and requires less rehab, but it's a little less strong. It would be a good choice for a middle-aged person with a moderate activity level who wants to take as little time off work as possible. The patellar tendon is often a better choice for large people with a more strenuous activity level—a college football player, for example—although they tend to cause more pain at the graft site and take a little longer to rehab.

An **allograft** uses tissue from somewhere other than the patient to rebuild the ACL. These grafts are often harvested from a tissue and organ donor, sterilized, and stored in a tissue bank until needed. Allografts have a high success rate, and are less traumatic since the tissue isn't taken from the patient.

Artificial synthetic grafts are also an option. In my opinion, they're not yet ideal for long-term success and strength, so I'd recommend the other two options first.

Discuss the two options with your surgeon. The pros of an allograft: there tends to be less pain, and the operation takes less time because there's no need to harvest the graft material from the patient. It's less invasive, and leaves fewer scars for the same reason. Allografts are your best bet if you've experienced patellofemoral problems in the past, if the original surgery didn't work, if you're having multiple ligaments reconstructed, or if your patellar tendon is very small. The downside: the very slim chance that the body will reject an allograft. These tend to be more expensive, have an extremely slim chance of disease transmission, and may be more prone to stretching and aren't as strong. Autografts, on the other hand, provide no concern for rejection or disease transmission but are associated with tendinitis in the graft site.

Most doctors prefer one procedure over another and become more proficient in that surgery. Barring other criteria, I'd go with the strength of your surgeon's preference.

Physical therapy. Surgery must always be followed by a program of physical therapy designed to restore proprioception, strength, and stability to the knee. Beginning physical therapy almost immediately after surgery has cut recovery times significantly. I recommend that patients do PT for at least four to six months following surgery; about two to three times a week for the first few months, and at least once a week after that, with supplemental "homework" exercises provided by your physical therapist or the workouts in Chapter 12 of this book.

How Long Will My Recovery Take?

Your speed of recovery depends on the degree of the injury, as well as your degree of commitment to the rehabilitation process. With proper strength training, you can be back to a full activity level after a Grade I sprain in four to eight weeks; and in eight to twelve after a Grade II sprain.

After surgery, you may bear weight on the leg immediately (unless your meniscus was also repaired) with assistance of brace and crutches, and you can usually return to sports within four to six months. Complete recovery, which means that you're back to your pre-surgical activity level, may take anywhere from six months to a year.

Rebecca Lobo, 29, *professional basketball player with the WNBA's Connecticut Sun*

"I blew my ACL in the first minute of the first game of the season in 1999. I knew it was an ACL as soon as it happened; it felt like a grenade had gone off in my knee. I'd never had a serious injury before that, and it was a difficult adjustment. I'm an athlete: it was the first time in my life that I couldn't just get up and go for a jog or a game of pickup whenever I felt like it— I couldn't even run across the street to beat a blinking "Don't Walk" sign. I did six months of rehab, but I re-tore the ACL that December, and spent the next two and a half years getting it healthy enough to play again. I was able to do recreational sports, but it took me a long, long time to get back to the very highest level, where I needed to be. I'm finally back to my preinjury condition, three and a half years later.

When I think about the time I spent rehabbing the second ACL, I wish I'd had a slightly healthier focus. Everything I did, every decision I made, was centered around my knee and getting it healthy enough to play. I remember the night of the Millennium, December 31, 1999. I didn't go to a party I'd been invited to, just in case someone who'd been drinking bumped into my leg—I'd just had surgery, and didn't want to take any risks. Now I think that may have been a mistake. Basketball is my life, my passion, and I love it, but there have to be other things as well. I was spending four hours a day in rehab, and that should have been enough. Part of the problem was that I'd just moved to New York to be close to my physical therapists, and while they were amazing, I might have been better off at home, with my friends and family around me, and other things to think about besides my knee.

*It's really hard to be patient, especially when you're a profes-
sional athlete and someone who's used to pushing yourself as hard
and as far as you can. You want all of your goals to happen in the
moment, but healing takes time, and you can't accelerate the
amount of time your body needs to get better. I think I was fully
healed the first time, but if I had it to do over again, I'd really
make sure. After I tore it the second time, my doctors and I took it
really slowly. Of course, I can understand the impulse to want to
get back to play as soon as possible. If you're a high school kid or
a college athlete, you want to make your next season, and all you
can see is the present. But you have to look at the bigger picture. I
want to be able to run around with my kids when I have them, and
I want to be able to go for a jog when I'm fifty. You've got to give
yourself the time to heal, and you have to understand that it's
about more than your next game—it's about getting yourself
healthy for life."*

THE POSTERIOR CRUCIATE LIGAMENT (PCL)

The PCL is the ligament in the inside of the knee joint, behind the ACL.
Its purpose is to prevent the lower leg from going too far back; when
something forces the lower leg farther back than the PCL can allow, this
ligament can stretch or tear, partially or completely. This happens less
often than an ACL tear, but more often than most people think.

How Can I Injure My PCL?

You can hurt your PCL by falling on your bent knee, or by sustaining
a serious impact to the front of the leg, forcing the lower leg backward.
The classic PCL injury is the "dashboard" injury, which happens when
the knee hits the dashboard. The PCL may also be damaged in the
course of other ligament injuries.

If you suspect that you've hurt your PCL, call your doctor. Anti-inflammatories and RICE may alleviate some of the pain before your visit.

HOW WILL I KNOW IF I HAVE A PCL INJURY?

Unlike the ACL, the PCL tends not to make a noise when it tears. Many of the other symptoms, including instability of the leg, swelling within the first two hours of the injury, and pain, are much less severe. In fact, there is often no swelling and it may feel like a minimal injury.

HOW WILL MY DOCTOR DIAGNOSE A PCL INJURY?

Your doctor will take a history of the injury and then do a physical exam to determine whether or not the PCL has been damaged. The physical exam will probably involve comparing your injured leg with the noninjured one to see if the lower injured leg sags and the classic PCL injury test, the posterior drawer test in which you lie on your back with your knees at 90 degrees. Your doctor will stabilize your foot and then push your shinbone toward you. If your PCL is damaged, your lower leg will move backward because it is no longer supported by the ligament.

Your doctor may also use MRIs and X rays to confirm the diagnosis and to determine whether there has been any associated damage to the cartilage and bone in the knee.

NON-SURGICAL TREATMENT OPTIONS

Treatment for PCL injuries tends to be determined by the severity of the injury and the likelihood that other components in the knee (cartilage, other ligaments, bone) are involved. If left untreated, a torn PCL may contribute to arthritis.

Minor, isolated PCL tears can usually be treated non-surgically. The natural healing history of isolated PCL injuries has long been debated, as many do very well when treated non-operatively. Most patients functionally adapt and tolerate a torn PCL for years, although it means an increased risk of osteoarthritis down the road.

RICE. Rest, ice, compression, and elevation combined with NSAIDs can help to alleviate the pain and speed healing.

Bracing. If you're planning on returning to a sport with a high risk of violent contact, like football or hockey, you may want to consider bracing your leg with a specially fitted hinged brace to give it additional support if someone crashes into it again.

Physical therapy. Physical therapy is recommended to strengthen the muscles around the knee, increase proprioception, and regain range of motion.

SURGICAL OPTIONS

If the patient is symptomatic and can't maintain stability in the leg, an isolated PCL tear may be surgically reconstructed. Surgery is often indicated when the PCL tear is combined with other ligament injuries.

PCL reconstruction. The PCL can be reconstructed using an autograft such as the patellar tendon or hamstring tendon, or an allograft.

Avulsion fracture repair. It is also not unusual for a completely torn PCL to take a piece of the shinbone with it; this is called an *avulsion fracture*, and will be picked up on an X ray. In this case, the ligament may need to be reattached to the bone using screws.

Physical therapy. Surgery must always be followed by a program of physical therapy designed to restore proprioception, strength, and stability to the knee, similar to the ACL Health Workout in this book.

WILL I RECOVER COMPLETELY, AND HOW LONG WILL IT TAKE?

You will be able to return to a fairly high level of athletic activity within four to six weeks without surgery and four to six months after surgery.

THE COLLATERAL LIGAMENTS

The two collateral ligaments are located at the inner and outer sides of the knee joint. The medial collateral ligament (MCL) connects the thighbone to the shinbone and stabilizes the inside of the knee. The lateral collateral ligament (LCL) connects the thighbone to the fibula, the smaller bone in the lower leg, and stabilizes the outside of the knee.

The collateral ligaments suffer damage when the lower leg is forced too far to either side.

THE MEDIAL COLLATERAL LIGAMENT

An MCL sprain or tear is one of the most common ligament injuries. It gets injured when the leg sustains force on the outside, forcing the foot out and the upper part of the lower leg in toward the other leg. It's often associated with sports like football, skiing, and soccer.

HOW CAN I INJURE MY MCL?

In football, the injury is usually the result of a contact blow to the outside of the leg while the foot is planted. In skiing, the force is put on the knee by the body itself. The foot slips outward, causing the body's full weight to come down on the unsupported inside of the knee. MCL injury can also be caused by sudden deceleration, twisting and pivoting, and cutting, as in soccer.

HOW WILL I KNOW IF I'VE INJURED MY MCL?

You may notice swelling or pain on the inside of the knee, accompanied by instability, or the inability to bear weight on the injured leg. In some cases, this does not happen immediately. You may find that it's difficult to get out of cars or to turn corners because of pain. You may find you can't sleep on your side with knees touching because of the pain—if this is the case, sleep with a pillow between your knees until the pain subsides.

HOW WILL MY DOCTOR DIAGNOSE AN MCL INJURY?

Your doctor will take a history of the injury and then do a physical exam to determine whether or not the MCL has been damaged. If your lower leg can bend outward more than normal, then you may have a tear in the ligament. This test is called the valgus stress test. See page 108 for an illustration of the valgus stress test.

Your doctor may also use MRIs and X rays to confirm the diagnosis and to determine whether there has been any associated damage to the cartilage and bone in the knee.

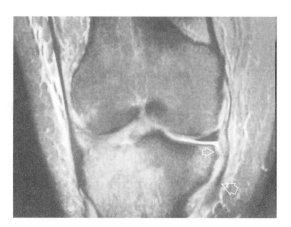

MRI OF TORN MCL

NON-SURGICAL TREATMENT OPTIONS

An isolated MCL, even a complete tear, most often heals nicely without need of surgery, but if other components of the knee have also been damaged, surgery may be indicated.

RICE. Rest, ice, compression, and elevation, combined with NSAIDs, can help to alleviate the pain and speed healing.

Bracing. Hinged bracing will protect against a load on the outside of the leg, but will allow full range of motion. Range of motion is essential: the normal stress you put on the ligament by bending and straightening it stimulates the collagen in the ligament to heal completely, without the detrimental stress of the valgus load. People with previous MCL injuries who want to continue activities may benefit from protective bracing to support the knee.

Physical therapy. Physical therapy is recommended to strengthen the muscles around the knee, increase proprioception, and regain range of motion.

Surgical Options

A very small percentage of patients will require surgical repair. The surgery involves reattachment or repair of the ligament and rehab.

Physical therapy. Surgery must always be followed by a program of physical therapy designed to restore proprioception, strength, and stability to the knee, like the General Knee Health Workout in Chapter 12 of this book with the exception of the inner thigh exercises.

Will I Recover Completely, and How Long Will It Take?

The MCL seems to recover faster and more fully than the ACL and PCL. Grade III MCL tears may require two to three months of rehabilitation before you can resume full activity.

The Lateral Collateral Ligament

The LCL keeps the outside of the knee stable. The LCL is injured much less frequently than the other ligaments in the leg.

How Can I Injure My LCL?

The mechanism of the injury is basically the reverse of an MCL sprain—the lower leg is forced inward, either by a twisting or pivoting motion, or a blow from an inside force. We see a lot of LCL sprains in sports that require a lot of sudden stop and turns, like basketball or soccer, and in sports where there is a lot of contact between players, like football and hockey.

How Will I Know If I Have an LCL Injury?

You may experience pain and swelling on the outside edge of the knee as well as a feeling of instability in the leg.

How Will My Doctor Diagnose an LCL Injury?

Your doctor will take a history of the injury and then do a physical exam to determine whether or not the LCL has been damaged. The physical exam will include bending your lower leg inward; if it bends inward more than normal, the ligament may be torn. This is the varus stress test. See page 109 for an illustration of the varus stress test.

Your doctor may also use MRIs and X rays to confirm the diagnosis and to determine whether there has been any associated damage to the cartilage and bone in the knee.

NON-SURGICAL TREATMENT OPTIONS

Isolated LCL tears usually heal nicely on their own. However, whatever injury caused the damage to the LCL probably damaged another ligament at the same time, so we rarely see an isolated LCL sprain. When the injury is isolated, or if the other injuries were also minor, these can usually be treated non-surgically. If the LCL is actually torn, partially or completely, with other ligament injuries, it may require surgical repair.

RICE. Rest, ice, compression, and elevation, combined with NSAIDs, can help to alleviate the pain and speed healing.

Bracing. People with previous LCL injuries who want to continue activities may benefit from protective bracing.

Physical therapy. Physical therapy is recommended to strengthen the muscles around the knee, increase proprioception, and regain range of motion. A full course of physical therapy for an LCL injury usually takes about three months.

SURGICAL OPTIONS

If you're considering surgery for an LCL injury, it's probably a complete tear and wasn't the only damage done to the knee. Rehab and surgery will have to do with the other injuries.

WILL I RECOVER COMPLETELY, AND HOW LONG WILL IT TAKE?

Isolated Grade III LCL tears may require two to three months of rehab before you can resume full activity.

INJURY TO ALL FOUR MAJOR LIGAMENTS

Severely traumatic incidents, such as a car crash or a serious sports injury, may result in tearing of several or all four of the major ligaments in the knee. This is also associated with total dislocation of the knee, and there may be associated vascular and nerve damage as well. Emergency care and surgery are indicated in these instances.

Meniscal Injuries

The menisci are the rubber washers of the knee. As you'll recall, there are two menisci in every knee: the C-shaped medial meniscus on the inside of the knee, and the semicircular lateral meniscus on the outside. The menisci are located at the center of the knee joint, and their primary function is to cushion the thighbone and to provide a smooth surface so that bone can glide across the shinbone instead of grinding against it. They also distribute forces across the knee and play a very important role in shock absorption.

The menisci are made of cartilage, a rubbery substance with limited blood diffusion. Some parts of the menisci have more blood vessels than other parts, which means that their ability to heal themselves varies, depending on the part of the cartilage that's hurt. In general, the outside of the meniscus is more likely to heal than the inside, where there are fewer blood vessels.

When we talk about meniscal injury, we're generally talking about meniscal tears, as the result of a trauma, overuse, or degeneration. And we're often talking about the medial meniscus, which is injured much more often than the lateral meniscus because of its unique anatomy. The medial meniscus is fixed to the walls of the capsule, so it's a sitting duck in the face of abnormal forces. The lateral meniscus, on the other hand, is fixed only on one side, so it has a little more play, and can more easily move around and out of harm's way.

There are a number of different kinds of meniscal tears, including the **bucket handle tear**, a tear in the inside rim of the medial meniscus, a **parrot beak tear**, and *fraying*, which is most often seen in cases of degeneration.

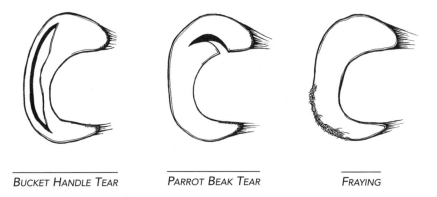

BUCKET HANDLE TEAR   PARROT BEAK TEAR   FRAYING

It's extremely common for meniscal tears to be associated with injuries to other components in the knee, especially ACL and MCL sprains and tears.

HOW CAN I INJURE MY MENISCUS?

The meniscus can be torn in the course of a traumatic incident, as part of an overuse injury, or as a function of degeneration in the knee.

Trauma. Any of the cuts, twists, pivots, sudden stops, or contact blows that can damage the ligaments in the knee can also tear the meniscus. These injuries often go hand in hand, and in some instances, the stretching of the ligament may actually be the force that tears the central cartilage. In some cases, the cartilage is torn by the knee snapping back into position after an inappropriate stretch—the meniscus gets caught in the hinge like a finger in a slammed door.

Overuse. The meniscus may also be damaged in a much more gradual way. Any repetitive compressive or rotational stress on the knee can cause the bones to grind up against the cartilage. Eventually it will begin to wear away, and little bits of the meniscus may be released into the joint, causing pain and swelling. Squatting or just bending the knee may tear the meniscus.

Degeneration. As we age, all the collagen in our bodies gets less flexible, and the cartilage in our knees is no exception. So when destructive chemicals are released into the joint as a result of arthritis, the cartilage is especially prone to erosion. Eventually, this will lead to fraying as the cartilage wears out.

HOW WILL I KNOW IF I HAVE A MENISCAL TEAR?

If you have a torn or damaged meniscus, you may feel pain and experience swelling in the knee. Whether you experience this pain and swelling on the inside or the outside of the knee depends on which piece of cartilage has torn, but it will almost certainly be along the joint line. Swelling and pain will probably not happen immediately (within a few hours) after the injury, but at some point over the next day. This may be followed by intermittent periods of swelling and pain.

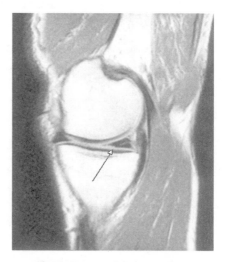

MRI OF MEDIAL MENISCAL TEAR

Usually, you have pain when you're going up or down stairs or squatting, and getting up from a low seat is often painful because of the compressive load placed on the meniscus. It may feel as if your knee is giving way.

You may experience the knee locking in position, or an inability to straighten or bend the knee past a certain degree. This happens when a piece of the cartilage breaks off and gets lodged in the hinge of the joint, preventing movement.

You may also hear a clicking sound when you move your knee, which is the sound of the cartilage moving against the bone in an abnormal way.

HOW WILL MY DOCTOR DIAGNOSE A MENISCAL TEAR?

Your doctor will take a history of the injury (if there was one) and then do a physical exam to determine whether or not the meniscus is damaged. The physical will include McMurray's test, where the ankle is turned while the leg is bent and straightened. This twists and compresses the meniscus, and the presence of pain, resistance, or clicking will alert your doctor to a tear. During the Apley test, you lie on your back with your knee flexed and your foot at a 90-degree angle to your body. If the meniscus is damaged, you will feel pain when downward pressure is applied to the foot. Pain is usually located over the joint line, either on the inside or the outside of the leg, and sometimes in the back. An MRI may be used to confirm the diagnosis.

NON-SURGICAL TREATMENT OPTIONS

Many small cartilage tears, especially those on the outer rim of the meniscus, can heal on their own. Even small meniscus tears that don't heal may become asymptomatic with rest and rehab.

There is no question that many mensical tears can become asymptomatic without surgery. In many cases, a damaged meniscus does not require surgery for a full recovery.

Calvin, 79

"I've been active my whole life, spending the majority of my career out in the field, which meant climbing up ladders and stacks. I've also been active in my personal life, doing a lot of biking, horseback riding, that kind of thing.

Last year, I sold my business, a business I had founded and managed for fifty years, and as you might imagine I was really down as a result. Then we went away for the whole summer, and I didn't bring any work with me, and I just had too much time to think. It was right around then that my right knee started to feel funny. I favored the other one for a while, but then it became clear that the pain wasn't to be ignored, so I went to the doctor and was diagnosed with a lateral meniscal tear.

The knee injury might be one way that my body was manifesting the stress I was feeling—maybe instead of getting an ulcer, I got a meniscal tear.

Things are better now. I'm working as a consultant at my old company, and the work is challenging and interesting. I'm not considering surgery. I'm wearing a simple knee sleeve and doing exercises to strengthen my legs, and I'm taking glucosamine. I'm also more sensible about the way I treat the joint, not getting myself into the silly positions I used to. When you climb up a ladder through a hatch and have to transfer your weight onto a platform, it's very hard to keep the load vertical. I have to figure out a way to do these things without taxing my knee. I go for long walks and bike rides, but I don't mountain climb. I'm not taking any pain medication at all.

I fully expect this to resolve eventually."

RICE. Rest, ice, compression, and elevation, combined with NSAIDs, can help to alleviate the pain and speed healing. Relative rest is especially important; putting too much pressure on a torn meniscus can cause further damage to the cartilage. Crutches are indicated for the first few days, until the pain abates. Ice and compression to quickly decrease the swelling allow earlier increased range of motion, which is a priority, taking care not to push too much flexion since this can cause pain. Forced flexion can put undue stress on the tear and delay healing.

Bracing. A knee sleeve or brace can help with compression and stabilize the knee while it heals.

Physical therapy. An exercise program designed to strengthen the muscles in the knee without putting undue pressure on the compromised meniscus is recommended. The Patellofemoral Health Workout in Chapter 12 is appropriate.

> **Note**: Sometimes an asymptomatic meniscal tear may flare up again. If this occurs, see your doctor for evaluation.

SURGICAL OPTIONS

If the tear is significant and causing pain, then surgery may be required, and since meniscal tears are so commonly associated with damage to the ligaments and other components in the knee, it's usual for the meniscus to be repaired or removed as part of a larger surgery. The goal of surgery should always be to leave as much of the meniscus intact as possible; risk of arthritis climbs when this protective cartilage is taken out of the knee. Different kinds of repairs are possible, depending on the size and type of the tear, and the location.

Suturing. Sometimes the tear can be repaired by sewing the two sides together, mending the tear.

Debridement/partial menisectomy. In this procedure, the part of the meniscus that has ripped is cut or shaved off. Any loose pieces of cartilage that have broken free are cleaned out of the joint, and the surface will be left smooth.

Total menisectomy. In some cases, when the meniscus has been damaged in a number of places and cannot be repaired, most of the meniscus has to be removed, but this is rare. When much of the meniscus is removed in the younger patient, meniscal transplant surgery should be considered to help prevent progressive deterioration and degeneration of the knee.

Meniscal transplant. Meniscal transplant surgery involves an allograft, which is harvested from a tissue and organ donor, sterilized, and stored in a tissue bank until it's needed. It's indicated for relatively young (under fifty) patients at a normal weight with no history of arthritis in the knee and stable ligaments.

HOW LONG WILL IT TAKE TO RECOVER?

Non-surgical. Small tears, especially on the outer rim, will heal themselves with rest in four to six weeks. I always recommend a program of physical therapy, most of which can be done on your own, to rebuild the strength in the muscles of the leg so you're not putting undue pressure on already compromised cartilage. The Patellofemoral Health Workout in Chapter 12 can be used.

Post-surgical. If you have surgery to trim or debride an isolated meniscus tear, you can generally be back at work within a week (as long as your job doesn't require manual labor). The length of your full recovery time depends on the type of surgery done and your compliance with physical therapy, but most people are active and pain-free in one to three months. Healing of the meniscus usually requires crutches for four to six weeks to protect the repair.

Physical therapy. After a short period of rest, the focus of rehabilitation is to strengthen the muscles around the knee. Your physical therapy program should include exercises like those found in my patellofemoral workout in Chapter 12.

MENISCAL TEARS AND ARTHRITIS

All knee injuries increase your risk of arthritis, but this is especially true with meniscal injury, which leaves the articular cartilage dangerously exposed to wear and tear. If parts of the meniscus are removed during surgery, this risk escalates and, the more meniscus that is removed, the more precipitously it escalates.

MENISCAL CYSTS

A meniscal cyst is a bag of fluid that sits on the joint line. It feels hard to the touch, and can be painful. Meniscal cysts usually accompany a torn meniscus, although there are rare instances of isolated cysts.

RICE, bracing, and NSAIDs can help to alleviate some of the pain. If the cyst does not subside on its own, it may need to be drained. If the cyst persists, the tear in the meniscus needs to be repaired or debrided.

DISCOID MENISCUS

When you're born, the meniscus is round. Most of the time, as you learn to walk, it evolves into the shape we ordinarily see, but sometimes, it doesn't evolve normally and you're left with that round meniscus—this is called a discoid meniscus.

You can go through life without ever knowing you have a discoid meniscus. The problem usually emerges (if ever) at preadolescence or adolescence. It isn't commonly a painful condition, but there may be a snapping noise when the child walks.

In some cases, this anatomical anomaly may cause a tear in the meniscus, with all the symptoms we've already discussed. Tears in a discoid meniscus are treated much the same way as a tear in a normal one, although if surgery is required, the surgeon may normalize the discoid shape to make the meniscus less prone to tears.

Tendons

The muscles are connected to the bones by extensions called the tendons. There are a lot of tendons in the leg, but four major tendons tend to present as knee problems: the quadriceps, the patellar, the iliotibial band, and the hamstring.

The most common tendon injuries are the result of overuse, although sudden ruptures resulting from trauma—getting hit, or a deep cut—are also a possibility. The major injuries of the tendons are:

- Tendinitis/tendinosis
- Osgood-Schlatter's disease
- Tendon rupture (patellar and quadriceps)
- Iliotibial band syndrome

Tendinitis vs. Tendinosis

You'll hear these terms a lot, and I want to straighten out any confusion there might be among them. Tendinitis is an inflammation of the tendon. It usually occurs as a result of some repetitive motion that causes the tendon to become inflamed when exercised beyond its normal capacity. When that injury continues to be irritated, it can cause a breakdown in the collagen, causing a more serious and chronic condition called tendinosis. Tendinopathy, incidentally, is a more general term spanning all different types of tendon injury.

TENDINITIS

An inflammation or irritation of any of the tendons in the knee is called tendinitis. One of the most common tendon injuries we see is patellar tendinitis, an inflammation or irritation of the patellar tendon, the largest and strongest single tendon of

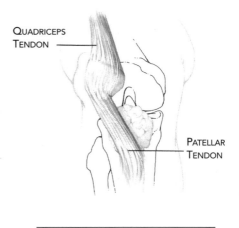

QUADRICEPS TENDON

PATELLAR TENDON

PATELLAR AND QUADRICEPS TENDONS

THE MOST COMMON KNEE PROBLEMS • 139

the knee. The quadriceps tendon and hamstring tendons are also prone to this condition.

How Can I Get Tendinitis?

Patellar tendinitis is also known as jumper's knee, because it is so often the result of jumping activities, such as basketball and volleyball. It's also found in runners, tennis, and soccer players because of the repetitive load they put on their tendons. Playing through pain and overexertion are two common contributors to the development of tendinitis in the knee.

How Will I Know If I Have Tendinitis?

You may experience pain in the front, back, or side of the knee when squatting, climbing stairs, or getting up from a chair. The area where the tendon inserts into the knee may swell, and it may be difficult to straighten or bend the leg. In the case of patellar tendinitis, it's common to find tenderness around or above the tibial tuberosity, the bony protrusion below the kneecap, where the patellar tendon joins the shinbone.

How Will My Doctor Diagnose Tendinitis?

Your doctor will probably be able to diagnose tendinitis during a comprehensive physical exam, especially if you experience pain when you're extending against forced resistance. An X ray may be used to rule out other problems, and an MRI may be used to confirm the diagnosis but should not be necessary.

Non-Surgical Treatment Options

If tendinitis is left untreated, it can make the tendon more vulnerable to rupture, or turn into the more serious tendinosis, which leads to even more chronic pain.

Usually, tendinitis can be treated conservatively, with an emphasis on relative rest. Eventually, the goal will be to strengthen and stretch the various muscle-tendon units to correct whatever caused the problem in the first place, but the first priority is to unload the knee.

RICE. Rest, ice, compression, and elevation, combined with NSAIDs, can help to alleviate the pain and speed healing.

Bracing. An *infrapatellar strap,* also called a counterforce brace, may help to relieve some of the stress on the patellar tendon by distributing pressure across the tendon. A knee compressive sleeve, available at a drugstore, can be used for added support, which may help reduce the swelling around the tendon.

Orthotics. If your doctor suspects that flatfeet caused the injury, he or she may suggest orthotics to correct the problem.

Ultrasound. High-frequency sound waves bounced off the injured area may increase blood supply, help with pain, and soften scar tissue. In a similar vein, shockwave therapy, which is similar to ultrasound, can be used.

Physical therapy. The focus of rehabilitation is to increase the flexibility and strength of the leg muscles. In addition, deep friction massage across the tendon can promote healing. Therapy should include exercises like those found in my Stretching Workout and the General Knee Health Workout in Chapter 12.

SURGICAL OPTIONS

In rare cases, surgical treatment is needed to treat tendinosis, when it is chronic and unresponsive for more than six months. In a procedure known as **patellar tendon debridement**, a small piece of the patellar tendon will be removed, in order to aid in healing the tendon.

HOW LONG WILL MY RECOVERY TAKE?

One to three months is generally enough time for a patient experiencing jumper's knee for the first time; if the condition is chronic, a flare-up may require a little longer before you return to full activity.

Post-surgical recovery takes about four to six months.

OSGOOD-SCHLATTER'S DISEASE

Osgood-Schlatter's disease is the condition commonly known as "growing pains." Growth plates are bands of cartilage that turn into bone as a child grows. There's a minor bony growth area in the knee right at the tibial tuberosity, the bony protrusion where the patellar tendon joins the shinbone. Children who engage in a lot of physical activity, especially running and jumping, are prone to the patellar tendon attachment on the shinbone becoming irritated and inflamed. It can even cause some elevation of the bone—in this stage of development, the tendon is actually stronger than the bone. In about 25 percent of cases, the condition is found in both legs. Once the bone fuses, the pain generally stops, although many children are left with an enlarged tibial tuberosity.

Osgood-Schlatter's disease is most common in physically active boys between thirteen and fifteen. Girls get it less often, and they tend to be a little younger if they do.

HOW WILL I KNOW I HAVE OSGOOD-SCHLATTER'S DISEASE?

You may experience pain, swelling, and sensitivity around the tibial tuberosity.

HOW WILL MY DOCTOR DIAGNOSE OSGOOD-SCHLATTER'S DISEASE?

The doctor will be able to tell if you have Osgood-Schlatter's after a physical exam, although he or she may order further tests to rule out other more serious problems, like a fracture or a tumor. An X ray may confirm that the bony area is larger than usual.

NON-SURGICAL TREATMENT OPTIONS

For the most part, Osgood-Schlatter's disease will go away of its own accord when the child stops growing, so there's no serious consequence to leaving this condition untreated. As a result, most treatments are actually targeted toward reducing the pain. An athlete should not be allowed to participate if he's limping on the field or court.

RICE. Rest, ice, compression, and elevation, combined with NSAIDs, can help to alleviate the pain and speed healing. Be sure to check the instructions on the box for the appropriate dosage, which may be different for an adolescent.

Physical therapy: After a short period of rest, an increase in hamstring flexibility and strengthening the muscles around the knee, especially the quadriceps, will help to prevent pain in the future. Therapy should include exercises like those found in my Patellofemoral Health Workout in Chapter 12.

Only in the most severe cases do we immobilize a patient with Osgood-Schlatter's, and only for a very short period of time—at most, a couple of weeks.

Surgical Options

In very rare cases, a piece of unfused bone may suddenly split from the growth area, essentially causing a fracture, and this may need to be surgically repaired.

How Long Will It Take to Recover?

A child may need to rest anywhere from three to six weeks, and may have to modify activities (avoiding deep knee bends, jumping, cutting, and sprints) to avoid pain. The pain almost always stops entirely after a short treatment or when the child stops growing—until that time, the pain may be intermittent. In many cases, the patient is left with an enlarged tibial tuberosity.

Tendon Rupture

A tendon rupture occurs when one of the major tendons rips, or rips completely away from the bone to which it's attached. This can be an extremely painful and debilitating injury; thankfully, it's relatively uncommon.

Although there are many tendons in the knee, the two most prone to rupture are the quadriceps tendon, which connects the quadriceps muscle to the patella, and the patellar tendon, which connects the patella to the shinbone. Patellar tendons are comparatively rare. Quadriceps tendon tears are most commonly found in people over forty; you may remember President Clinton undergoing surgery to treat this injury in 1997.

HOW CAN I RUPTURE A TENDON?

This usually occurs as the result of a trauma, but may also be a consequence of leaving tendinitis untreated. It was standard practice to repeatedly inject cortisone into a painful tendon site, but we now know that this can lead to tendon rupture; if you had this treatment in the past, you're at higher risk. Do not allow anyone to inject your patellar tendon. People who suffer from rheumatoid arthritis are also at higher risk.

HOW WILL I KNOW I HAVE A RUPTURED TENDON?

You will be unable to straighten, fully extend, or bear weight on the injured leg.

HOW WILL MY DOCTOR DIAGNOSE A RUPTURED TENDON?

Your doctor will take the history of the injury and do a full physical exam. Usually, he'll be able to feel a gap where the tendon is supposed to be.

On an X ray, the kneecap will often appear out of position (higher than usual if the patellar tendon is ruptured; lower than usual if the quadriceps tendon is ruptured). An MRI may be necessary to confirm the diagnosis.

TREATMENT OPTIONS

If the tendon has been completely ruptured, it must be repaired surgically; the tendon will be sewn back onto the bone. The surgery cannot be done arthroscopically.

Physical therapy. Surgery must be followed by a physical therapy program designed to restore proprioception, strength, and stability to the knee. I recommend that patients do PT for at least six months following surgery: about two to three times a week for the first few months, and once a week after that, with supplemental "homework" exercises provided by your physical therapist or those in this book.

HOW LONG WILL MY RECOVERY TAKE?

After surgery to repair a ruptured tendon, you're going to be in a cast or brace for about six weeks. It may take up to six months before you're able to perform your full activities.

ILIOTIBIAL BAND SYNDROME

The iliotibial band is a muscle-tendon combination package, and it stretches all the way down the outside of your leg, from your ilium (your pelvis) to your tibia. When the leg moves, the IT band moves over the outside bump, or condyle, at the bottom of the femur; the repeated rubbing of the band over the bone can cause the irritation of the bursa there, which causes pain.

Iliotibial band syndrome is common among runners and cyclists because of the repetitive nature of these activities. It's often found as a result of overtraining, weakness, and a lack of flexibility in the iliotibial band itself, running on crowned surfaces (or always in the same direction on a track), and anatomical irregularities, such as leg-length discrepancy and flatfeet.

HOW WILL I KNOW I HAVE ILIOTIBIAL BAND SYNDROME?

The outside of your knee will hurt, often in a general area, as opposed to one specific spot. Your leg may creak as you flex and extend it. You may also feel pain below the knee, where the band inserts into the shinbone, or in the thigh and hip. The pain may be worse after activity, especially running downhill or climbing up and down stairs. Walking with stiff legs may alleviate the pain, because it doesn't permit the IT band to rub against the bone.

HOW WILL MY DOCTOR DIAGNOSE ILIOTIBIAL BAND SYNDROME?

Your doctor will do a complete physical examination, including a series of tests designed specifically to diagnose iliotibial band syndrome. One of the tests is to hold the bony knob on the outside of the bottom of your femur while bending and straightening your knee. If you feel pain at 30 degrees, that's a sign that the iliotibial band is sliding over the bone, which is causing iliotibial band syndrome. Your doctor may also test the tightness of your iliotibial band by moving your leg across your body while you're lying on your back or on your side. Additional imaging isn't usually necessary.

TREATMENT OPTIONS

Iliotibial band syndrome can almost always be treated conservatively. Although there is a surgical procedure to release the band slightly, it's almost never necessary, and I rarely recommend it to my patients.

RICE. Rest, ice, compression, and elevation, combined with NSAIDs, can help to alleviate the pain and speed healing. Icing after activity may especially help.

Physical therapy. After a short period of rest, stretching and strengthening the band itself as well as the gluteus muscles will help to prevent pain in the future. Therapy should include exercises like those found in my Patellofemoral Health Workout in Chapter 12. Stretching and strengthening the hip abductors and flexors and correcting whatever training problems caused the problem in the first place are the two single most important ingredients in treatment and preventing reinjury.

Cortisone injections. An injection of anti-inflammatory medication may help to reduce swelling and pain. This can be used for recalcitrant cases. We try not to inject the tendon directly but instead the area around the tendon, and to avoid repeated injections.

Bursa

The bursa are small, protective, fluid-filled sacs found all over the body, often where the tendons connect to the bones. These can become inflamed if irritated, a condition called bursitis. If the inflammation is chronic, the tissue around the bursa may harden. The irritated bursa may also become infected.

The most commonly injured bursae are the ***prepatellar*** bursa, the ***pes anserinus*** bursa, and the ***infrapatellar*** bursa. The prepatellar bursa is literally in front of the patella. The pes anserinus bursa is located about two inches below the kneecap, on the inside of the leg, where the three parts of the hamstring muscle connect to the shinbone; when inflamed, the three tendons look like the foot of a goose, which explains how pes anserine bursitis gets its name: *pes anserinus* means "foot of the goose" in Latin, and the condition is regularly referred to goosefoot bursitis as a result. The infrapatellar bursa is located under and just below the kneecap.

HOW DO I GET BURSITIS?

There are several ways to irritate the bursa. One is trauma: you can fall directly on, or get hit on one of the bursa. This causes bleeding into the sac, which will swell. This is often seen in combination with another traumatic injury, like an injured tendon. Another common cause is overuse, especially with prepatellar bursitis, which is also known as "housemaid's knee," because it is associated with kneeling. It's often seen among people whose occupations force them to spend a lot of time on their knees: roofers, carpet layers, plumbers, etc. Recreational gardeners may also experience this condition.

How Will I Know If I Have Bursitis?

You'll experience pain and swelling over the bursa, especially after activity. In the case of prepatellar bursitis, this will be in the area directly over the kneecap; with pes anserinus bursitis, it will be toward the inside of the leg. You may also feel a lumpy area in the skin over the kneecap. Inflamed bursa can become infected, which makes this condition very serious. Signs of infection include your knee becoming hot, red, very swollen and tender, and you may experience a fever.

How Will My Doctor Diagnose Bursitis?

Your doctor will diagnose bursitis through a physical examination. If she suspects an infection, she may insert a needle and remove some fluid for testing.

Non-Surgical Treatment Options

This injury is one that can usually be treated conservatively. With rest, the fluid in the bursa will be absorbed back into the body, and the swelling will recede.

RICE. Rest, ice, compression, and elevation, combined with NSAIDs, can help to alleviate the pain and speed healing. Avoid any activities that irritate the knee.

Aspiration. If the swelling is slow to abate, or if your doctor suspects an infection, she may insert a needle into the bursa and drain some of the fluid in it.

Antibiotics. If the bursa is infected, you'll be put on a course of antibiotics.

Cortisone injection. If there is no sign of infection, your doctor may inject the anti-inflammatory medicine cortisone into the bursa to help reduce the swelling and pain.

Knee pads. If your occupation or recreational activity requires you to spend a lot of time kneeling, you should consider using knee pads as a preventive measure when you're ready to go back to it. A compressive knee sleeve may help to decrease the swelling.

SURGICAL OPTIONS

In rare cases, surgery is necessary to remove a bursa that has thickened so that it is interfering with your ability to move. The bursa may grow back.

HOW LONG WILL MY RECOVERY TAKE?

After surgery, you'll need to stay off your feet for a week, but you should be back to all activities in two months.

POPLITEAL (BAKER'S) CYST

Baker's cysts are benign tumors found in the back of the knee, caused when the popliteal bursa fills with fluid.

HOW DID I DEVELOP A BAKER'S CYST?

These cysts are often the result of excess fluid building up in the knee, often as the result of another inflammatory knee condition. Arthritis is the most common culprit, but cysts also commonly occur with chronic meniscal tears. Sometimes they develop in adolescents without any underlying cause.

HOW WILL I KNOW IF I HAVE A BAKER'S CYST?

There will be a swollen bump on the back of your knee. You may have diffi-culty straightening or bending the knee completely. If the cyst is irritated, you may experience pain, either during activity or all the time. If it ruptures, your lower leg may swell and become painful.

HOW WILL MY DOCTOR KNOW THAT I HAVE A BAKER'S CYST?

Your doctor will determine that you have a Baker's cyst through a physical examination. An ultrasound or MRI may be used to confirm the diagnosis. If the cyst ruptures, the condition looks very much like a more serious condition called thrombophlebitis, a blood clot in a swollen vein. Your doctor will make sure that you don't have thrombophlebitis with a special test that uses sound waves called a venous Doppler.

NON-SURGICAL TREATMENT OPTIONS

Unless the cyst is causing you pain or disfigurement, your doctor may suggest a conservative approach. Many of these cysts resolve on their own. The best way to treat them is to address their underlying causes, such as the arthritis causing the swelling.

RICE. Since the cyst is caused by swelling in the knee, controlling the swelling is an important first step to resolving it. Compressing the knee while icing it and taking NSAIDs may help to reduce swelling.

Cortisone injections. If you're not having any luck with ice and the NSAIDs, corticosteroids are more powerful anti-inflammatory agents that can be injected directly into the joint, reducing pain and swelling. I don't recommend cortisone injections more than two to three times a year.

Aspiration. If the swelling is not going down, a needle may be inserted into the joint to withdraw some of the fluid causing it. You can also directly aspirate the cyst. The use of ultrasound as a visual aid is often helpful for this procedure.

SURGICAL OPTIONS

If the cyst is causing pain or threatening to compress one of the veins in the back of the leg, it can be addressed surgically. If you do decide to have the cyst removed, the procedure is relatively simple: an incision is made, the cyst is removed, and the wound is stitched. More often than not, if you address the underlying cause of the knee swelling, the cyst will resolve on its own.

How Long Will My Recovery Take?

You may be off your leg for about one week, but should be back to activities within a few months.

Bone/Articular Cartilage

There are four major bones in and around the knee: the femur, or thighbone; the tibia, or shinbone; the fibula; and the patella, or kneecap. These provide structure, stability, and strength for the leg.

Stress Fracture

A stress fracture is one of the most common sports injuries, most often the result of overuse. More than 50 percent occur in the lower leg. Stress fractures that cause knee pain can happen in the thighbone, shinbone, and in the kneecap itself.

To understand why a stress fracture happens, first you have to understand the way bone works. Bone is living tissue, and it renews itself. In the same way exercise breaks down your muscles so they can come back stronger, you have to break down your bone so it can rebuild. In other words, the bone responds to stress by shedding the old bone and making new bone in its place; the bone gets stronger to support the load. This is why we advise people at risk for osteoporosis to walk and do other forms of weight-bearing exercise.

If there's too much stress, though, the bone can't keep up. The degeneration is faster than the regeneration, and the resulting discrepancy leads to a stress fracture. Thus activities that cause too much stress without the appropriate amount of time for the bone to build puts you at risk. Starting an exercise program at a vigorous level, for instance, puts you at high risk; the bone hasn't had the chance to strengthen itself before being put under a great deal of pressure.

Some people have stronger bones than others. This is a combination of genetics and lifestyle—someone who ran in high school is more often going to have stronger bones than someone who didn't. And someone who's been taking a calcium supplement since adolescence will probably have better bone strength than someone who starts in their thirties—or their fifties. I recommend that my female patients consume 1500 mg of calcium, and 400 I.U. of vitamin D a day in order to keep their bones strong, either through their diet or in supplement form. It's also important to wear proper running shoes that provide an adequate amount of cushioning.

CHANGE YOUR SHOES!

The ability of a running shoe to absorb shock decreases with every mile you run. Running shoes that don't offer adequate cushioning play a significant role in your risk of developing a stress fracture. You should replace your shoes every 250 to 400 miles. Replace them more often if you run a lot, or if you have a high arch, a little less often if you run less than 30 miles a week.

Women get stress fractures more often than men do. They often have less muscle mass to absorb shock, and they can be at higher risk if they have a condition called "the female athlete triad," a combination of an eating disorder like bulimia or anorexia combined with an infrequent or absent menstrual cycle and bone loss.

HOW WILL MY DOCTOR KNOW IF I HAVE A STRESS FRACTURE?

Your doctor will suspect a stress fracture by your description of the symptoms and a physical examination of your leg. An X ray may be used

to confirm the diagnosis, but if the fracture is caught early enough, it may not show up on the X ray. Microfractures or swelling in the bone may appear on an MRI. In the past, a bone scan was the gold standard, but an MRI is just as sensitive and does not have the radiation exposure that a bone scan has.

Nancy, 33

"I had gotten out of a very long, bad relationship, and my self-confidence was in the toilet. A running buddy who was training for her eighth marathon talked me into training with her, arguing that it would be just the thing to distract me from my broken heart. She was right: setting goals and meeting them was good for my self-esteem, and the grueling training schedule certainly took my mind off my ex-boyfriend.

I'd run a lot and was already in good shape, but there wasn't really enough time to get ready for a whole marathon—or rather, enough time for my bones to get ready. Often, toward the end of my training sessions, I'd notice a little pain in my kneecap, but I iced it and ignored it. Once or twice, when it got bad, I'd take a couple of days off, and it would get better.

The day of the marathon arrived, and I thought I was in fighting shape. It was a gorgeous day, perfect running weather, and I felt really strong. But around mile 15, that pain in my knee was starting to nag at me. Around mile 20, it was actively hurting. And at mile 24, I was limping, just barely able to use it at all.

I finished the marathon—and in so doing, I finished the stress fracture I'd apparently been working on for a couple of months. Over the twenty-six miles, I'd taken a hairline fracture to completion. I spent the next six weeks in a knee immobilizer, and the next four months in rehab. Now, I tell everyone who will listen: don't train through pain! And warming up is more than a five-minute jog at the beginning of your workout—you have to do a couple of months of "warm-up" before you do something major like a marathon."

WHAT ARE MY TREATMENT OPTIONS?

RICE. Rest, ice, compression, and elevation can help to alleviate the pain and speed healing. Tylenol or a similar pain medicine can be used for pain as opposed to the NSAIDs, which may delay bone healing. In more minor fractures, relative rest may be enough to allow the bone to heal after a short period of immobilization; in more severe cases, the bone must be immobilized for six to eight weeks in a brace.

Bone stimulation. Bone stimulators, which send an electrical current through the bone, can be effective for fractures that are slow to heal. They're not a first line of treatment, however.

Physical therapy. After a period of relative rest, a physical therapy program designed to strengthen the muscles around the knee and to build bone strength is recommended, one like my General Knee Health Workout in Chapter 12. It's essential to hold off on returning to high-impact activity until your doctor assures you that the bone has healed completely, or the process will simply begin again.

Surgery. Rarely required to set the bone in place.

HOW LONG WILL IT TAKE TO RECOVER?

Your recovery time depends largely on the degree of the fracture. In the case of a severe, completed stress fracture, the bone may take up to six months to heal.

OSTEOCHONDRITIS DISSECANS

This occurs when a piece or pieces of articular cartilage and the bone that it's attached to separate, either partially or completely, from the rest of the bone. This usually happens in the medial femoral condyle—the inside bump at the bottom of the thighbone—but it can also occur in the lateral, or outside condyle and in the patella. The loose pieces of cartilage and bone, called loose bodies or "joint mice," can get trapped in the joint and cause locking and pain, and the uncushioned bones rubbing up against each other can also cause pain—and eventually arthritis.

HOW DO I GET OSTEOCHONDRITIS DISSECANS?

Osteochondritis Dissecans (OCD) happens because the blood supply to the bone has become compromised. We're not entirely sure why this happens. Some cases occur after trauma. Other theories include an unnoticed injury, a genetic predisposition, or a growth disturbance, since it seems to happen most often among adolescents and young adults. It happens most in athletes, especially young men, although we're now seeing more cases in active girls.

HOW WILL I KNOW IF I HAVE OSTEOCHONDRITIS DISSECANS?

Your knee will hurt, especially after activity, and there may be some swelling. The knee may also catch or lock when extended or bent, and it may be difficult to fully extend the leg. You may feel more comfortable walking with your lower leg rotated outward, because that takes the pressure off the inside condyle.

HOW WILL MY DOCTOR KNOW IF I HAVE OSTEOCHRONDRITIS DISSECANS?

If the lesion is on your medial femoral condyle, the inside of your knee will be tender at about 30 degrees of flexion. Your doctor may also do an X ray to see if the bone shows signs of damage, and an MRI may be necessary to determine whether

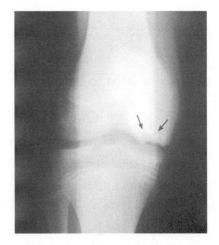

X-RAY OF OCD

or not the bone and cartilage are still attached or loose in the joint.

Occasionally your doctor will spot what we call "silent" or asymptomatic OCD on an X ray while looking for something else. If this isn't causing you any discomfort, and you're young enough that we can expect a reasonable healing response, you may simply be monitored.

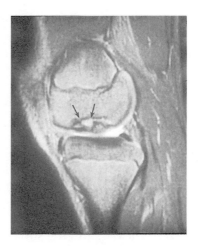

MRI OF OCD

NON-SURGICAL TREATMENT OPTIONS

If the bone and cartilage fragment are stable, that is, if they are still attached and not loose in the joint, conservative treatment can be attempted. This is especially true for younger people. It is important for this condition to be treated if it's symptomatic. Once the articular cartilage has been compromised, there's nothing to protect the bone, and this can easily lead to arthritis.

Immobilization. A short period (up to six weeks) of relative immobilization is recommended so that the bone can get a jump start on the healing process, combined with unloading weight on the leg through the use of crutches. Then we suggest that you modify activity for one to three months, so that you're not doing anything that causes pain.

Physical therapy. A physical therapy program designed to strengthen the muscles around the knee without putting undue pressure on the injured bone and cartilage is recommended, one like the General Knee Health Workout in Chapter 12.

Bracing. A knee sleeve or brace can help with compression and stabilizes the knee while it heals. A brace that unloads stress from one side or another of the knee may also be helpful.

SURGICAL OPTIONS

If conservative treatment doesn't work, if the fragment is unstable, or if the patient is older, surgery may be indicated. Surgical procedures used to treat OCD are generally done arthroscopically and are designed to restore a smooth surface to the bone and the cartilage. The fragment may need to be anchored to the bone, loose bodies will be removed, and the surface of the bone may be abraded to stimulate regrowth. Bone grafts, either from the patient or a cadaver, may be considered.

Cartilage cell transplant. If there has been significant damage to the cartilage, your doctor may recommend replacing it. There are a number of ways that cartilage can be replaced, all of them relatively new and experimental. In a relatively new procedure, called a *biological knee replacement*, your surgeon will harvest the body's own articular cartilage and bone, mash it up into a paste, and apply that paste to a spot on the bone that has no articular cartilage of its own because of degeneration. This procedure can be done arthroscopically. A bone covered with undamaged articular cartilage can also be harvested from a non-weight-bearing area in the body and implanted. Alternatively, cartilage cells can be harvested from the patient and grown in a laboratory into healthy cartilage, which can then be implanted into the joint.

Because the cells come from your own body, they're not rejected by the body (although in some cases, it is necessary to use donated tissue).

Physical therapy. A physical therapy program designed to gradually strengthen the muscles around the knee and gradually increase bone strength without putting undue strain on the healing fracture is recommended. My General Knee Health Workout, done without pain, is recommended.

OSTEONECROSIS OF THE KNEE

Also called avascular necrosis, osteonecrosis, which means "bone death," has much in common with osteochondritis dissecans. It occurs when a piece of the bone loses its blood supply and begins to die, and it also most commonly occurs in the medial femoral condyle (it may also occur on the outside of the leg or on the surface of the shinbone). It begins as a problem isolated to the bone, although it may ultimately result in involvement of the cartilage and osteochronditis dissecans.

It is most commonly seen in women over sixty, and is three times more likely to happen in women than in men.

HOW WOULD I GET OSTEONECROSIS?

Like OCD, we're not exactly sure how this condition develops. An undiagnosed injury may cause an altered blood supply. Osteonecrosis of the knee is also associated with certain conditions and treatments, such as obesity, sickle cell anemia, lupus, kidney transplants, and steroid therapy. It has also been linked to decompression problems among deep-sea divers.

HOW DO I KNOW IF I HAVE OSTEONECROSIS?

You may have pain and swelling on the inside of the knee, especially after activity.

HOW WILL MY DOCTOR KNOW IF I HAVE OSTEONECROSIS?

Your doctor may suspect osteonecrosis based on your description of the symptoms and a physical exam, but the diagnosis is really made with an MRI or bone scan. It has to be at a fairly advanced stage before it begins showing up on an X ray.

NON-SURGICAL TREATMENT OPTIONS

Conservative treatment is appropriate in the early stages of the disease. It cannot be ignored: if left untreated, this disease can cause severe osteoarthritis and the complete collapse of the bone.

RICE. Rest, ice, compression, and elevation can help to alleviate the pain and swelling. Calcitonin, a hormone nasal spray that slows down bone reabsorption, can also help with pain and might aid in healing. Crutches should be used to unload the knee.

Bracing. A knee sleeve or brace can help to stabilize the knee.

Physical therapy. A physical therapy program designed to strengthen the muscles around the knee without putting undue pressure on the injured bone and cartilage is recommended, such as my General Knee Health Workout in Chapter 12.

SURGICAL OPTIONS

If a substantial amount of the bone area is affected (usually more than half), your doctor may recommend surgery. Several different procedures may be used to treat osteonecrosis of the knee, including debridement, where any loose pieces of cartilage and bone that have broken free are cleaned out of the joint and the surface left smooth; or drilling to hollow the bone in order to reduce pressure on the bone surface.

Bone grafts, either from your own body or from donors, may help to support the knee while the damaged bone heals. Osteotomy, a procedure in which the surgeon removes a wedge-shaped piece of bone from one side of the shin or thighbone to compensate for the degeneration on the other side of the leg, can change the alignment of the leg by altering the place the load is borne. In severe cases, those that have resulted in advanced osteoarthritis, a total knee replacement may be required.

Arthritis

The word "arthritis" comes from the Latin *arthro-*, which means joint, and *–itis*, which means inflammation—literally, "inflammation of the joint." This inflammation is the result of deteriorated articular cartilage, the slippery cushion at the end of the bones that works to absorb shock and facilitate easy movement of the bones over each another. As this cartilage wears down, bone rubs against bone, causing swelling and pain. Fragments of bone and cartilage may break off, causing further pain and interfering with the ability of the joint to move, and bone spurs may form as part of the body's attempt to repair itself. Inflammation may also result from some autoimmune disorders.

You can get arthritis in any joint in the body; here we'll be dealing with it as it pertains to the knee. As far as I'm concerned, arthritis is the greatest threat to knee health in this country today. With the graying of America and the rise in active seniors, I've seen the number of arthritis sufferers in my own practice skyrocket over the last ten years. The high rate of knee injury in middle-aged people means that those numbers are only going to continue to increase.

There are over 100 different types of arthritis, caused by as many different factors—including gout, lupus, and viral hepatitis. The majority of the patients I see fall into two categories, those with *osteoarthritis* or *rheumatoid arthritis*. Osteoarthritis is by far the most common: the Arthritis Foundation estimates that the disease affects approximately 20.7 million people in the United States. Rheumatoid arthritis affects 2.1 million Americans, mostly women.

Unfortunately, there is no cure for arthritis. But that doesn't mean you're condemned to a life of chronic pain. With the proper care and treatment, it is possible to live actively and well with this disease. In this section, I'll outline the differences between the types of arthritis and give you some tips as to how you can make your arthritis accommodate your life—not the other way around.

OSTEOARTHRITIS

Osteoarthritis, or OA, is not only the most prevalent form of arthritis, it's the most commonly seen joint disease. Also known as degenerative, or wear-and-tear arthritis, it's generally seen in people forty-five and older, and women suffer from it more commonly than men do. The knee is the most commonly affected joint.

What causes osteoarthritis? Like most late-onset diseases, it's a combination of genetics and lifestyle. You may be genetically predisposed to arthritis, or you may have inherited certain anatomical irregularities, such as the alignment issues we discussed in Chapter 3, which leave you vulnerable to this disease. People who are bow-legged or knock-kneed are more likely to develop arthritis, for instance.

Those whose occupations require heavy manual labor, and people whose recreational activities are extremely vigorous do put more strain on their joints over the course of their life, and that leaves them at higher risk. A previous knee injury of any kind—especially a ligament injury that has left the joint unstable, a meniscus injury, patellar dislocation, or osteochondritis dissecans—will also leave you more vulnerable to post-traumatic arthritis.

One of the single largest contributing factors—to the onset of arthritis and to the rapid development of the disease once you have it—is carrying excess body weight. **I tell every single one of my arthritic patients to lose weight if they need to.**

How WILL I KNOW THAT I HAVE OSTEOARTHRITIS?

You will experience pain, aching, and stiffness in your knee, especially in the morning, or after sitting for a while. Activity may be painful, and pain may be worse after you've stopped moving. You'll notice that your range of motion is compromised. You may experience crepitus, a crunching sound or feeling when you move the knee, and the joint may be swollen and tender.

You may also find that your knee has turned into a more reliable weather predictor than television. All of our joints have nerve endings that are sensitive to pressure changes, which may be one reason an arthritic joint aches before a rainstorm. The damaged or painful joint may be more sensitive to the drop in pressure.

How Will My Doctor Know If I Have Osteoarthritis?

Your doctor will listen to your symptoms, watch the way you walk, and perform a physical exam. There's no blood test for osteoarthritis, but a blood test will help your doctor to rule out other kinds of arthritis. An X ray will help to confirm the diagnosis of osteoarthritis; on the X ray, you may see that the space between the bones has gotten smaller, and any changes in the bone itself (like a spur) will show up.

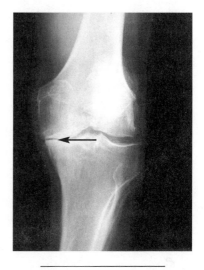

X-RAY OF OSTEOARTHRITIS

What Are My Treatment Options?

Osteoarthritis has no cure, but that doesn't mean it can't be treated. In fact, there are many treatment options for you to discuss with your doctor. These include protecting your joints, as well as using medication, exercise, taking comfort measures to increase your comfort, and maintaining your normal activity level to slow the progress of the disease. Let's explore some of these options together.

Protect Your Joints

It stands to reason that the less wear and tear you put on the joint, the slower the degeneration. We don't want you to stop moving under any circumstances, so you need to think about ways you can make movement more comfortable.

Weight loss. As soon as I've diagnosed overweight patients with arthritis, I start talking to them about ways they can manage their weight. Even a small weight loss can make a substantial difference in slowing the disease's progression and the amount of pain felt. (See the weight loss tips on pages 53-55 for more information about ways you can lose the excess weight and protect your knees from further damage.)

Switch activities. You don't have to stop working out, but you may have to modify your activity level—and what you do. A general rule of thumb: if it hurts, don't do it. You've got nothing to gain from "working through pain" with OA, except further damage to your cartilage. Luckily, many activities can give you a good workout without punishing your knees. Consider moving from a joint-impact sport like basketball or running to one that's a little more forgiving on the joints, like cycling or swimming. You'll find more information on low-impact exercise on pages 62-64.

Lifestyle modifications. Look around you. Is there anything you can do to make life a little easier for your knees?

Whenever possible, avoid unnecessary activities like climbing stairs and heavy lifting. For instance, many of my patients, even those with only moderate symptoms, have experienced a great deal of relief by moving their bedroom to the first floor of their home. You may want to invest in a set of bar stools with backs so you don't have so far to go when you're sitting down on or standing up from a chair. There are any number of products specifically designed to help a person with arthritis live more comfortably, from a device that can help you open jars to elevated toilet seats. Use them! (The Arthritis Foundation *www.arthritis.org* provides a list of easy-to-use products on their website.) You'll not only be happier, but you'll be saving your joints some wear and tear.

Orthotics. Shoes or shoe inserts that have lots of cushioning reduce the amount of shock and stress going across the knee. If your arthritis was caused by an anatomical irregularity (people with flatfeet often develop arthritis in the inside of the knee, for instance), it's not too late to protect the joint from further distress by investigating an orthotic insert to correct the anatomical problem.

Use walking aids. A cane or a walker takes pressure off the injured joint and may help you keep active without pain. If walking is your primary form of exercise, try to walk on a cushioned, forgiving surface, like grass or a track instead of concrete. Wear shoes that provide good cushioning and support.

Bracing. A knee sleeve, available from a drugstore, may provide additional support, warmth, and stability. Unloading knee braces can help people to walk and exercise without pain—talk to your doctor about exploring this possibility.

MEDICATION

The assumption that we've been making thus far about medications has been that you'll use them for a short period of time in the case of a traumatic injury, or intermittently, in the case of overuse injuries—say, when you feel pain after activity.

Obviously, people who are living with chronic pain have a different set of criteria. There's no hard and fast rule of thumb for how often you should take medication: That's something you're going to have to decide with your doctor, based on your level of pain and the success of other comfort measures. I will say this: all medications have side effects, and the less you take, the less likely you are to experience those side effects. My rule of thumb for my own patients is to: take as few drugs as you can, in as low as dose as you possibly can, while still managing the pain. Explore other measures for controlling the pain whenever possible. If you need to take medications on an ongoing basis, please make sure that this is done under the supervision of your doctor.

Topical creams. Creams, rubs, and sprays, many of which are available over-the-counter, may help. Some creams contain salicylates, the leading ingredient in aspirin, which is something to be mindful of if you're taking aspirin (you may want to use the cream and the pills on alternate days).

Others include capsaicin, which is the ingredient that makes chili peppers hot. It heats the skin and actually blocks a chemical that delivers pain messages to the brain. It needs to be rubbed into the skin a number of times a day, and you may have to use this cream for a week or more before noticing significant improvement. Wash your hands very carefully before touching your eyes, and make sure that no cream gets into an open cut.

You may experience some minor skin irritation with some of these products—if a rash develops or the irritation persists, you'll want to stop using the cream. These should not be used in combination with heat or under a bandage.

Acetaminophen (Tylenol). Although Tylenol isn't an anti-inflammatory, a number of convincing studies have shown that it's even more effective than some of the over-the-counter anti-inflammatories in controlling arthritis pain. In fact, it's the only drug that many of my patients use, although you can also talk to your doctor about the possibility of combining it with one of the NSAIDs.

NSAIDs. The non-steroidal anti-inflammatory drugs (both the over-the-counter kind, like ibuprofen, aspirin, and naproxen, and the prescription kind—the Cox-1 and Cox-2 inhibitors, like diclofenac and celexocib) that are discussed in Chapter 2 may help to reduce the inflammation in the joint and provide pain relief.

If you're taking NSAIDs on a regular basis, you should be getting regular screening blood tests (blood count, kidney and liver function) every three to four months.

Cortisone injections. If you're not having any luck with acetaminophen or the NSAIDs, corticosteroids are more powerful anti-inflammatory agents that can be injected directly into the joint, reducing pain and swelling. I don't recommend cortisone injections more than two to three times a year; there's evidence that repeated injections actually contribute to the degenerative process. Oral corticosteroids are not used to treat OA.

Viscosupplementation. Hyaluronic Acid Treatment (*Synvisc, Hyalgan*) is a relatively new injection treatment (it was approved by the FDA in 1997), that requires a series of three to five injections over the course of a month, done in your doctor's office. It's actually not a drug: hyaluronic acid is manufactured by the body and is present in healthy joints. The injections merely supplement your natural supply, which is depleted in OA patients. The injections don't cure the disease, but they do reduce pain and stiffness for six to eight months in most patients.

These injections tend to be fairly well tolerated. In rare cases, there is an increase in swelling and knee pain a day or two after the injection, but it's usually temporary and can be tolerated if you stay off your feet and take acetaminophen or an NSAID. Since some of these medications are derived from rooster combs, they should not be taken by anyone allergic to chicken or chicken products.

I've had a lot of success with this treatment. It's especially good for people who don't have advanced arthritis, but I've seen it do a surprising amount for people with a severe form of the disease as well. It doesn't work for everyone, but if it does work, it lasts six months to a year. One of my patients couldn't walk three holes on the golf course before his pain drove him onto the cart. I did a single series of Synvisc on his knees, and four years later, he walks 18 holes five days a week. I'm not sure if the hyaluronic acid is still working, or if the exercise is actually the treatment, but one thing is clear: the Synvisc allowed him to get that exercise in the first place.

Violet, 67

"The problem with my knees started at birth. I'm a little bowlegged, and I hyperpronate. I was a very active person. I ran five miles a day every day, and would regularly join my husband, a foreman of a construction company that renovates brownstones, to routinely carry eighty-pound bags of concrete up and down flights of stairs. In other words, I really pushed the envelope on my joints.

I think that even if I'd known what I was doing, I would have kept it up—I was working for the security of my family. Anyway, by the time I was sixty, I'd completely destroyed my feet, my knees, and my lower back. I was diagnosed with tears in the meniscus in both knees in 1997, so I went in for surgery to have those taken care of. While they were in there, they confirmed that I had fairly advanced chondromalacia, so they did some smoothing.

All of this surgical stuff was just buying time. I knew it, and the surgeon knew it. I went to physical therapy, and hated every second of it. They handed me over to a twenty-year-old girl who acted as if we were going to be jumping out of an airplane together behind enemy lines, and you just can't do that to me. Every time I left there, I felt like I should be leaving in an ambulette. I didn't know any better; I thought that was just what it was supposed to be like, so I quit.

Anyway, the meniscus surgeries didn't do much to relieve the pain in any kind of permanent way, and soon I was pretty much back to where I'd started. I'd been hearing and reading about these Synvisc treatments, so I started asking around. I know a lot of doctors socially, including a retired orthopedic surgeon, and he pooh-poohed me, saying it was a fad and wouldn't work. My own doctor at the time gave me 101 reasons why he wouldn't recommend it, none of which made any sense to me. I think he thought I was going to deprive him of a knee replacement surgery. So I kept digging and asking around.

I eventually found a younger doctor who thought the injections were just the ticket for me. My insurance company wouldn't pay for it—they called it "experimental," but I was willing to pay for it myself if it meant relief from this pain. We did a series on both of my knees, and the results were completely miraculous. I felt better, more pain-free than I had in years. And I started at another physical therapy place, recommended by my new doctor, and the experience has been like night and day. The treatment is age- and condition-appropriate. I don't feel abandoned—there's none of this "Do one hundred of these and I'll be back when you're done." I've been doing a lot of work there to strengthen the inside of my leg so the muscle on the outside isn't dragging my kneecap all over the place and destroying the cartilage underneath.

The great results from the Synvisc lasted for about a year. This winter, I started to experience symptoms again and went back for another course. This time, it worked on my left leg but not on the right. At the same time, I got X rayed, and my doctor told me that the right leg had taken another step down. So that leg is still in a lot of pain, even when I'm at rest, and walking more than a few city blocks is almost more than I can bear. To make matters worse, the prescription NSAID I was on made my blood pressure skyrocket, so I can't even get any relief that way.

I told my husband that I'm getting sick and tired of being sick and tired. I can't live like this—when you get passive, you just get old. I want my life back. I want to be able to live normally without pain. So now I have an appointment with a surgeon to talk about the possibility of a knee replacement. I'm anxious about it. I

*hate how invasive the procedure sounds, and the commitment that
you have to make to physical therapy is heavy-duty—it's going to
be like having a job. I want to make sure that there's no less-inva-
sive treatment option out there before I pursue this, but I'm not
going to live like this anymore.*

*I'm deeply grateful to the Synvisc—it bought me a lot of time.
I'm glad I pursued it, even when all the advice I was getting was
steering me away from it."*

Glucosamine and chondroitin sulfate. These are dietary supplements, taken orally, that may relieve the pain of osteoarthritis. They
have helped a great number of my patients, and I suggest that you read
more about them in Chapter 13 on complementary medicine.

EXERCISE

Move—*even if you don't want to*. It's the easiest thing in the world to
let arthritis dictate what you will and won't do. But it's essential that
you keep moving, for a number of reasons.

First of all, stretching and exercise designed to increase your range
of motion will help with the pain you experience as a result of
osteoarthritis. The first issue on the agenda is to work on flexibility
across the knee joint. When we're in pain, we have a tendency to
"splint" ourselves—we instinctively immobilize the joint ourselves in
order to protect it. While this does protect us from pain in the short-
term, it causes tightness and contraction—and more pain—over the
long haul. Increasing flexibility and range of motion is ultimately very
beneficial. Gaining strength in the muscles that support the knee will
also help to relieve some of the pain you feel as you remove some of
the stress across the joint. It will also help to keep the joint healthy.

The benefits of exercise don't stop there. It's not news that we experience pain subjectively. We're all familiar with the stories of football
players who are so caught up in the competitive spirit that they don't

realize they're playing with a fracture, for instance. There's a lot of evidence that arthritis patients who exercise experience less pain and depression as a result of their condition than those who don't.

This may have something to do with the natural endorphins that are released when we exercise. The increased range of motion and strength that exercise buys arthritis sufferers also allows them to continue with their activities of daily living, which is a good feeling in itself—you feel better because you can do more. When you're actively participating in your care, you have an increased sense of control: the feeling that you're on top of the disease, as opposed to being a victim of it.

The answer might be a combination of all of the above—or none of them—but I notice an enormous and positive increase in the psychological well-being and physical state of my arthritis patients who exercise regularly.

That said, it's important to remind you of the essential balance between exercise and rest. If you're tired, or if your joint is tired and especially swollen or irritated, listen to your body and take a break. I'm still not recommending complete immobility—there's nothing wrong with a few gentle range-of-motion exercises as long as they're not causing you pain—but you can save the harder stuff for a day when you feel better. Again, please don't "push through the pain." While I can't promise that you won't feel a twinge or two, when exercise is seriously painful, it's a message from your body that you're causing additional damage.

COMFORT MEASURES

Ice. Ice will obviously help with the swelling you may experience, and you may find it physically soothing as well.

Heat. I don't recommend heat for most knee injuries because it can increase the amount of blood in the joint and promotes swelling.

Arthritis is the big exception. Because heat allows the muscle tissues to relax, it eases stiffness, and can be a real gift to the arthritic.

Some ways you can use heat:

— Take a hot shower in the morning.

— Soak in a hot bath; if you have access to a whirlpool or a Jacuzzi, you may find the movement of the hot water soothing.

— Apply moist hot packs directly to the sore area.

— Apply heating pad or hot water bottle.

— Contrast hot and cold. Use ice packs and heating pads alternately: thirty seconds of ice, followed by a minute of heat, followed by thirty seconds of ice, repeating the cycle for ten minutes.

  Some guidelines for using heat: hotter isn't necessarily better. The warmth should feel good, not uncomfortable. Never fall asleep with a heating pad on or you run the risk of waking up with a nasty burn. Use heat the way you would ice: apply for twenty minutes, leave it alone for an hour, heat for another twenty minutes. When you remove the heat source, your skin should be pink and warm, not red, mottled, hot, or blistered, and it should return to its normal appearance in half an hour or so. Don't ever combine heat with a topical cream like capsaicin.

Talk about it. We've discussed the importance of attitude in dealing with a chronic disease such as arthritis. One of the things that can dramatically improve your outlook is the ability to talk about your experience.

The more support you have, the easier it is to keep your spirits up. If you don't have friends and family close by, consider other options in your community. Even if you have a good support system, you may also want to look into the possibility of joining an arthritis support group— it can help to talk to people who know first-hand what you're going through. The Arthritis Foundation (**www.arthritis.org**) has local offices that can refer you to resources in your area, and you may find their extensive message boards a welcoming community.

Murray, 46

"My right kneecap was shattered in a car accident fifteen years ago. It healed OK, although it was always a little stiffer than the other one. About two years ago, I started experiencing pain in the knee, and it went from painful to excruciating in record time. My doctor told me I had arthritis.

You could have knocked me over with a feather. I was forty-two years old! I'd always thought that arthritis was something that happened to older people. And when he broke the news to me that there was no cure, I took it really hard.

I knew that I had to protect my joints if I was going to make it to a ripe old age on this knee, and I really thought that meant living in a bubble. All I could think about was the stuff I wasn't going to be able to do—the skiing vacation I take with my college buddies and their families every year, hiking and picnicking with my wife, even just lifting our toddler seemed incredibly dangerous.

I was totally unprepared for what it's like to live with chronic pain. It hurt all the time! I was so scared that the disease would progress really rapidly, leaving me crippled, that I basically cut down on physical activity altogether. I think I was also eating (and drinking) more because I was depressed. As a result, I gained about twenty-two pounds, which made the situation even worse. I felt bad about the way I looked, I felt bloated and weak physically for the first time in my life—and since my father died of early heart disease, I knew that I was putting myself in the way of a speeding train. Plus, I was doing exactly what I'd been trying to avoid in the first place by putting more stress on my knee.

After about a year of this, my wife had had enough. She went over my head and talked to my doctor about what was going on. He'd noticed the weight gain, but I hadn't mentioned the depression or anything else, so he didn't know I'd been taking the diag-

nosis so hard. I'm not really the support group type, but it did help to acknowledge the depression and the impact that the diagnosis had made on me. He was also able to talk to me a little about low-impact exercise and some pain management techniques that went beyond the Tylenol I'd been eating by the handful.

I've been much healthier over the last couple of months, and I feel much better. I haven't lost all the weight I'd gained, but I've lost about half of it, and that's helped my mood and my knees. I feel much better now that I'm exercising again. My wife has been amazing throughout this, and has really helped me to factor this disease into my life without letting it take over. She bought us both bikes for my birthday, so that's what we do together on the weekends now.

The only advice I can give to people who are diagnosed with arthritis is this: it is a big deal, and it does change your life, and it can be really terrifying and isolating, especially if you don't deal with it. But if you don't deal with it, your body gets worse, and so does your state of mind. Talk to someone in your life or your doctor if you think you're getting depressed, and get some help."

We'll discuss more comfort measures in Complementary Medicine, Chapter 13.

Surgical Options

If your OA is especially advanced and causing you such a tremendous amount of pain that you're unable to continue with activities of daily living, and no conservative remedies have helped to alleviate your pain, your doctor may suggest a surgical treatment.

Note: Unlike other surgical treatments discussed in this book, surgeries to treat arthritis are generally not permanent solutions. I've provided some general guidelines for the longevity of these procedures, but the results strongly depend on a number of factors, including the way the procedure is done and your level of activity. You should always ask your doctor or surgeon how long you can expect to reap the benefits of a procedure before you undergo it.

Debridement. As the bone and cartilage wear down, pieces may break off, causing pain by getting caught in the joint. This procedure, which is done arthroscopically, flushes those loose pieces out. Your surgeon may repair torn cartilage while he's in there, and rough the bone with an abrasive, which may encourage the growth of new cartilage. If the procedure is successful, you may experience relief from symptoms for a few years.

Proximal tibial osteotomy. Most osteoarthritis affects the inside of the leg. As the inside of the joint wears down, the lower leg becomes bowlegged. This further exacerbates the problem. Because of the anatomical shift, you're putting more pressure on the inside of the knee, which speeds the degeneration, which makes you more bowlegged—you get the picture.

A proximal tibial osteotomy corrects this malalignment; the surgeon removes a triangular piece of bone from the outside of the shinbone to compensate for the degeneration on the inside of the leg. In other words, you go from being bowlegged to normal, or even slightly knock-kneed. Unfortunately, the degenerative process in the inside of the leg begins again, so your relief from symptoms will probably last only about five to ten years, depending on your level of activity.

It's heavy-duty surgery. Expect your leg to be immobilized in a cast or a splint for four to eight weeks; it may take up to a year for you to regain a normal activity level. This procedure is usually considered the last line of defense before a total knee replacement, and is usually done in active people under sixty.

Unicompartmental joint replacement. Also called a partial knee replacement, this surgery replaces one part, or compartment of the knee instead of the entire joint. It's less invasive than a total knee replacement and requires less time to heal, but it is used only if the arthritis is isolated to one side of the joint.

Total knee replacement. This is an option for people who have not responded to any other type of treatment. Although it really is the surgery of last resort, its results last longer. As you can probably tell from the name, it involves the complete replacement of the knee joint with an artificial one, usually made of metal, plastic, and ceramic. Your surgeon will make a cut in your leg to expose and open the knee joint completely. The surgeon will remove the ends of your thigh and knee bones, and glue artificial bone ends in their place.

The joints last up to twenty years; surgeons are often reluctant to consider this surgery in people under sixty because they're more likely to "outlive their joint" and require another replacement (called a revision), which is harder to do successfully the second time around. Younger people are also more active and tend to wear the joint out much faster than the elderly.

A new surgery for knee replacement requires a much smaller incision, but early reports seem to indicate that it's harder to get the kind of precise fit that's

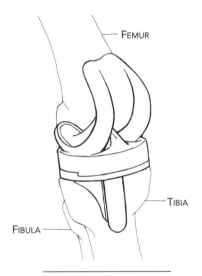

TOTAL KNEE REPLACEMENT

so important for a successful outcome. Talk to your doctor about this option.

Cartilage grafts. There are a number of ways that cartilage can be replaced. In a relatively new procedure, called a biological knee replacement, your surgeon will harvest the body's own articular cartilage and bone, mash it up into a paste, and apply that paste to a spot on the bone that has no articular cartilage of its own because of degeneration. This procedure can be done arthroscopically. A bone covered with undamaged articular cartilage can also be harvested from a non-weight-bearing area in the body and implanted. Alternatively, cartilage cells can be harvested from the patient and grown in a laboratory into healthy cartilage, which can then be implanted into the joint.

Because the cells come from your own body, they're not rejected by the body (although in some cases, it is necessary to use donated tissue). These procedures, still considered relatively experimental, are usually done in more active, younger people who have not yet experienced a serious degree of degeneration as a result of their OA.

RHEUMATOID ARTHRITIS

Rheumatoid arthritis is an autoimmune disease, which is to say that it happens when the body's immune system turns against itself. It cannot be cured, but there are treatments to slow the progression of the disease and reduce pain.

As you'll remember from Chapter 3, the anatomy chapter, the knee is encased in the synovium, a capsule filled with fluid that lubricates the moving parts in the knee and brings important nourishment to the parts within the capsule.

For some reason, rheumatoid arthritis causes the body's natural defense against infection to turn against the synovium. White blood cells, ordinarily responsible for attacking infections, go after the cartilage and bone. The synovial lining responds by swelling, and the muscles and ligaments that surround the knee are weakened and damaged.

We're not sure why rheumatoid arthritis happens: some people appear to be genetically predisposed, and researchers think that there may be environmental and hormonal triggers as well. A study published in the *Journal of Rheumatology* in 1999 indicated that smokers of cigars and cigarettes were at a 50 percent higher risk for rheumatoid arthritis—yet another good reason to quit!

RA tends to occur in people between twenty and forty-five, but it's also found in the elderly and in children. It seems that the later the disease appears, the less severe the symptoms. It is *three* times as likely to appear in women as in men.

RHEUMATOID ARTHRITIS AND BONE LOSS

People with rheumatoid arthritis are at especially high risk for osteoporosis, a condition that causes bone loss, leaving bones brittle, weak, and prone to fracture. This is especially true if you've been taking oral corticosteroids to help with your RA. Women are at special risk, since their chance of developing osteoporosis increases as they age and go through menopause.

In 2001, the American College of Rheumatology developed the following guidelines to help people who take corticosteroids minimize their risk for developing osteoporosis:

— Take the lowest possible effective dose of corticosteroids.

— Have a bone mineral density test before you begin taking the corticosteroids.

— If you smoke, quit.

— Limit your alcohol consumption.

— Try to exercise for between 30 to 60 minutes a day. Concentrate especially on weight-bearing, low-impact exercise, as that's the best way to build bone. For more information about low-impact exercise, see pages 62-64.

You'll also want to talk to your doctor about taking calcium and vitamin D supplements, and I recommend that my female patients with rheumatoid arthritis and osteoporosis take Fosamax or Actonel, two prescription medications that can improve bone density.

HOW WILL I KNOW IF I HAVE RHEUMATOID ARTHRITIS?

As with other types of arthritis, you'll feel pain, achiness, and stiffness in the affected joint. The symptoms of rheumatoid arthritis do differ from those for osteoarthritis, however. Unlike osteoarthritis, the stiffness you feel in the morning lasts more than half an hour. The joint may feel warm and tender to the touch. Rheumatoid arthritis tends to be symmetrical.

You may also experience systemic symptoms, such as a sense of fatigue or a feeling of general unwellness called malaise. You may develop a fever. Anemia, neck pain, and bumps under the skin near the joints (known as rheumatoid nodules) may also accompany this disease.

Your symptoms may not be consistent over a long period of time. Some people have symptoms for only a couple of months before the disease abates on its own. In most people, the disease flares up periodically, giving them serious symptoms for a period of time. In rare cases, this disease goes into remission.

HOW WILL MY DOCTOR KNOW IF I HAVE RHEUMATOID ARTHRITIS?

Because the symptoms present in different ways in different people, and because there's no one definitive test, RA can be difficult to diagnose. Your doctor may test your blood for something called "rheumatoid factor," which indicates you may have the disease. Although not everybody tests positive for this antibody, its presence occurs in 80 to 90 percent of people with RA. (Its presence may also indicate another autoimmune disease.) Your doctor may also perform a sedimentation rate test, which measures how fast red blood cells settle in the bottom of a test tube, and can alert us to the presence of inflammation.

An X ray will tell your doctor if there has been damage to your bones, and how much. The X ray changes in rheumatoid arthritis are much different from those in osteoarthritis.

NON-SURGICAL TREATMENT OPTIONS

There's no cure for rheumatoid arthritis, but there are a number of strategies you can adopt to make you more comfortable, some of which may actually slow the progression of the disease.

Rest. Although immobilizing the joint will lead to muscle atrophy and increased pain, it's important to rest when you're tired, or when the disease is active and the joint is actively swollen and painful.

Ice. Some patients find that icing the painful area helps; some do not. It can help to reduce the swelling, which is beneficial.

Exercise. The actress Kathleen Turner has rheumatoid arthritis, and in an interview with HealthTalk Interactive (*www.healthtalk.com*) about the disease, she said that her own personal breakthrough with the disease took place about five years after her diagnosis. She went to a new doctor, and he said, "Get into a pool every day. However much it hurts, however tired you are, get into the pool and swim as long as you can stand it."

I might not go that far with it, but I am a firm believer that people with rheumatoid arthritis should do as much exercise as they possibly can, for many of the reasons we've discussed already vis-à-vis osteoarthritis. To sum up: exercise will help alleviate pain; increasing range of motion counteracts our instinctive urge to "splint" or immobilize a joint that hurts, an urge that hurts us more over the long term; and strengthening the muscles that support the damaged knees will help with the pain of RA. Moving the joint itself is beneficial and prevents loss of function, and enables you to continue with your regular daily activities longer. The endorphins from exercise are a terrific way to combat depression and anxiety, and it will help you feel that you have control over the disease.

Remember, it's important to get adequate rest. People with RA are prone to fatigue and should always pay attention when their bodies tell them to slow down.

MEDICATIONS

NSAIDs. The non-steroidal anti-inflammatory drugs (both the over-the-counter kind, like ibuprofen, aspirin, and naproxen, and the prescription kinds like indomethacin and meloxicam) that are discussed in Chapter 2 may help to reduce the inflammation in the joint and are used by almost all patients with RA.

Remember, all NSAIDs come with a risk of side effects, especially fluid retention, potential ulcers, increased blood pressure, gastrointestinal distress, and kidney damage. If you're taking these on a regular basis, it should be under a physician's supervision, and your blood should be tested regularly.

Corticosteroids. Oral corticosteroids like prednisone may help to reduce inflammation, and there is some evidence that, in low doses, they may actually help to reduce the likelihood of joint damage. These drugs do have a number of problems associated with them, however. For instance, people often gain weight when they're taking them—never a good thing for your knees. Plus, when you stop taking them, they stop working; the pain returns and the disease continues to progress. In fact, because these drugs mimic one of the body's natural hormones, the body stops manufacturing that hormone, often leaving you worse off than you were when you started treatment.

Considering that the drugs also have negative long-term side effects, like an increased risk of bone loss, eye cataracts, and diabetes, the decision to begin oral steroids can be a difficult one. The higher the dosage, the greater the risk that you'll experience side effects.

Disease Modifying Anti-Rheumatic Drugs (DMARDs). How soon your doctor will put you on these medications depends on his or her personal strategy for dealing with this disease. Degeneration in the joint can happen very early in its natural course—sometimes after a few months. Many doctors will wait until more conservative therapies, like NSAIDs, have failed to control the swelling and the pain; others will put you on DMARDs immediately after diagnosing you with rheumatic arthritis in an attempt to cut off degeneration at the pass. Over the last year, rheumatologists have recognized the importance of starting these DMARDs early in the course of treatment.

DMARDs are slow-acting, which is to say that you may be on them for several months before you start noticing a difference in the way you feel (as opposed to the NSAIDs and steroids, which take effect immediately). Fortunately, these drugs can be used in combination with the NSAIDs.

The most commonly used DMARD is methotrexate, which suppresses an overactive immune system (it was originally used as a chemotherapeutic drug). This drug is generally taken in pill form, once a week, and can cause nausea, headache, dizziness, sensitivity to the sun, and a loss of appetite. Taking folic acid may help to alleviate some of those side effects, but you should talk to your doctor about dosages before you combine any supplement with medication. More serious side effects include a higher instance of liver disease, so your liver function should be carefully monitored if you're on methotrexate.

Other commonly used DMARDs include sulfasalazine (*Azulfidine*) and antimalarial drugs, like hydroxychloroquine sulfate (*Plaquenil*). Leflunomide (*Arava*) was developed especially for RA. All of these drugs have side effects ranging from the annoying (nausea, diarrhea) to the severe (liver and eye disease, other infections, and death). As with all medications, their use must be carefully monitored by a doctor.

Biologic response modifiers. These new rheumatoid arthritis medications (*Enbrel, Remicade, Humira, Anakinra*), work to control inflammation. They control symptoms of RA and may actually stop the degeneration in the joint. They're expensive, and must be injected once or twice a week (you can do this yourself). *Remicade* is taken less frequently, but must be infused through an IV in a hospital or doctor's office.

These drugs seem to be fairly well tolerated, but side effects may include an infection or irritation at the site of the injection, and more serious opportunistic infections can lead to death. You should be checked for infections such as tuberculosis before taking some of these drugs. Enbrel has been linked to nervous system disorders like multiple sclerosis, seizures, and the inflammation of the nerves around the eyes. Talk to your doctor about side effects before you begin taking this medication. These drugs should be discontinued if you develop an infection, and should always be taken under the close supervision of a physician.

SURGICAL OPTIONS

Total knee replacement. A total knee replacement is an option for people who have not responded to any other type of treatment; it really is the surgery of last resort and involves the complete replacement of the knee joint with an artificial one, usually made of metal, plastic, and ceramic.

The joints last up to twenty years; surgeons are often reluctant to consider this surgery in people under sixty because they're more likely to "outlive their joint" and require another replacement (called a revision), which is harder to do successfully the second time around. Younger people are also more active, and tend to wear the joint out much faster than the elderly.

Synovectomy. This is a rarely performed arthroscopic procedure, where parts of the inflamed synovium are actually removed. It's not all that effective, mostly because not all of the damaged tissue can be removed, and the synovium may grow back. It's most commonly done in combination with another surgical procedure, like a tendon reconstruction.

The Patellofemoral Joint

The patella is the kneecap, which rides on top of the knee joint. It's a small, oval-shaped bone, which moves so your leg can move, gliding up and down in a triangular-shaped groove cut into the femur, called the *trochlear groove*.

Although we refer to the knee as a joint, it's actually made up of a few of them, and one of them is the patellofemoral joint, or the place where the kneecap intersects with the bottom of the thigh-bone. Because this part of the knee experiences a tremendous amount of the load that is transferred across the knee (about half your body weight when you're walking on a flat surface, about five times when you're walking up stairs, and eight times your body weight when you're getting up from a chair without using the arms), it is a common source of anterior knee pain.

The patellofemoral joint can experience various problems. The first is that the patella, like any bone, can be fractured. Other problems occur when the patella isn't sliding smoothly within the center of the trochlear groove. This is called a tracking problem. If the bone is putting undue stress on one side or another of the groove, or on the cartilage beneath it, then it's creating patellofemoral syndrome, which can in turn damage the cartilage underneath the patella, causing chondromalacia. Sometimes the patella actually jumps out of the groove. If it jumps the track entirely, that's a dislocation. If it moves out of place and jumps back, that's called subluxation.

PATELLOFEMORAL SYNDROME AND CHONDROMALACIA

Patellofemoral syndrome is what happens when the patella, or kneecap, rubs against the bottom of the thighbone instead of moving smoothly across it. This can happen in one or both knees. The result can be a gradual wearing down of the articular cartilage at the end of that bone. This is called **chondromalacia**, and it leaves you at higher risk for arthritis.

I'd like to sort out some confusion concerning the two terms. Chondromalacia literally means the softening of articular cartilage of the knee. This is a potential pre-arthritic condition. Unfortunately, this has become a catch-all term, often used to describe general anterior knee pain, even when there's no damage to the cartilage at all. I call general anterior knee pain patellofemoral syndrome, or patellofemoral stress syndrome. If there is damage to the articular cartilage, that's chondromalacia.

Eventually, if patellofemoral syndrome is allowed to progress uncorrected and untreated, it can lead to chondromalacia, but the two terms cannot and should not be used interchangeably.

HOW DOES PATELLOFEMORAL SYNDROME DEVELOP?

Patellofemoral syndrome is often an overuse injury—specifically, the overuse of a joint that may or may not have anatomical abnormalities, like uncorrected pronation, an overly wide Q angle, miserable malalignment, or knock-knees. If you're stronger in the outside part of your quadriceps than you are in your inner quads, then the discrepancy may cause tracking problems with the patella—those stronger muscles on the outside of your leg will keep dragging the kneecap off course, causing irritation of the patella.

Patellofemoral syndrome can be associated with an extremely tight system of supporting soft tissue on the outside of the leg, called the *lateral retinaculum*, and/or with extremely tight hamstrings. When you have one of these abnormalities and overuse the joint, you're likely to develop stress in the patellofemoral area. Being overweight is another common cause of patellofemoral pain and chondromalacia.

We see patellofemoral syndrome a lot in athletes who place a great deal of repetitive stress across the knee—runners experience this condition so often that it's been nicknamed "runner's knee," and it's often seen in skiers as well. It may also be the result of trauma—a blow to the knee that causes the patella to rip off a piece of the articular cartilage, or a piece of the cartilage and the bone itself. This is called an osteochondral fracture.

In general, patellofemoral syndrome is found in more women than men. We especially see a lot of patellofemoral syndrome among young female athletes. During growth spurts, the pressure on their knees increases, as well as any anatomical irregularities that can exacerbate this condition, such as an increased Q angle and knock-knees.

How Will I Know If I Have Patellofemoral Syndrome?

You will feel a pain under or around the front of the kneecap. It may be worse when you are performing activities that involve bending, like squatting, or that involve lunging forward, like walking down stairs or a hill. You may also be stiff with knee pain after you've been sitting for a long time, a condition we call "theater knee."

In some cases of chondromalacia, you will actually be able to hear the bones grinding together when the leg is straightened and flexed. The symptoms you experience will vary according to the degree and type of damage to your cartilage.

How Will My Doctor Diagnose Patellofemoral Syndrome?

Your doctor will diagnose patellofemoral syndrome from your history, the location of the pain, your alignment, and the rest of your physical exam, which will probably include a number of tests to determine how mobile your patella is and how painful it is when compressed.

An X ray may be used to confirm that there are no other problems in the knee causing your pain, as well as looking at how the patella sits in the trochlear groove. An MRI may be used to see exactly where the articular cartilage under the patella is damaged.

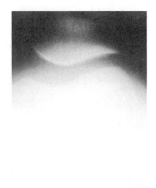

X-RAY OF NORMAL PATELLA

A true diagnosis of chondromalacia can take place only following an MRI or arthroscopy that determines softening of the articular cartilage, but it is not necessary to get a true diagnosis to treat this condition.

NON-SURGICAL TREATMENT OPTIONS

Most patients with patellofemoral syndrome can be treated conservatively and you should stick with this treatment, if necessary, for long periods of time. Because of the risk that this condition may turn into more serious conditions like chondromalacia and eventually osteoarthritis—and because it's painful, it is essential not to ignore it!

X-RAY OF SUBLUXED PATELLA

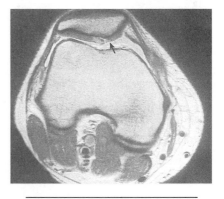

RICE. Rest, ice, compression, and elevation, combined with NSAIDs, can help to alleviate the

MRI OF CHONDROMALACIA PATELLA

pain and speed healing. Avoid the activities that cause you pain. Icing after activity may help and you'll want to limit squat, lunges, stairs, and flexion extension machines. You're putting the least pressure possible on your patellofemoral joint when your knee is straight or just partially bent, so in the interests of resting the joint and avoiding irritation, you may want to keep the leg relatively straight while you're resting.

Bracing. A knee sleeve or brace can help with compression and to stabilize the kneecap while it heals. Your doctor may recommend a patellar stabilizing brace, which has a C-shape, U-shape, or donut-shape pad that encourages your knee to track properly.

Patella taping. Literally taping the patella in place seems to alleviate pain during activity, although it doesn't always stop the patella from moving around. Some physical therapists have stopped using this technique, called McConnell taping, because it's time-consuming, but it can relieve pain. If you do pursue taping, you should be taught to tape yourself by a knowledgeable physical therapist, trainer, or physician.

Physical therapy. A physical therapy program designed to strengthen the quadriceps, especially the VMO, and stretch the hamstring muscles in the knee without putting undue pressure on the patellofemoral joint is recommended. Most of these can and should be done independently. You'll find an appropriate Patellofemoral Health Workout in Chapter 12 of this book. This is the mainstay of treatment for this very common disorder.

Glucosamine and chondroiten sulfate. If your doctor suspects that your patellofemoral syndrome has or is threatening your articular cartilage, you may want to have a discussion with them about the possibility of beginning these two supplements.

SURGICAL OPTIONS

If fragments of articular cartilage are loose in the joint and causing it to lock, your doctor can perform an arthroscopic procedure to

rinse those fragments out and smooth the remaining articular cartilage so that it's less prone to further damage. If your patellofemoral
syndrome is chronic and resistant to physical therapy, your doctor
may recommend surgery to correct the anatomical imbalance causing
the problem.

Lateral release. If the cause of your patellofemoral pain might be
a tight lateral retinaculum—and if this condition is resistant to
conservative treatments such as a rigorous stretching program—your
doctor may recommend an arthroscopic procedure called a lateral
release.

In this procedure, the lateral retinaculum is cut and released,
which relieves some of the pressure on the kneecap and allows it to
return to proper tracking in the trochlear groove. Eventually the ligaments that have been cut heal, and scar tissue fills in the gap left by
the surgery. Sometimes the tendons on the inside of the leg need to
be tightened as well.

Many people, myself included, think that the lateral release is
overused. I really prefer for my patients to try orthotics, strengthening and stretching for a while before I recommend this procedure.
Most patients do not need surgery for this disorder.

For more serious problems, especially if they're accompanied by
partial or complete dislocation of the patella, more serious open
surgery may be required to reposition the patella, usually by changing the place where the patellar tendon, which attaches the kneecap
to the shinbone, is attached.

Debridement. If you have chondromalacia, small bits of the articular cartilage may have worn off to get trapped in the joint, causing
pain and locking. If this is the case, your doctor may recommend an
arthroscopic procedure done to smooth out the uneven cartilage and
rinse the cartilage fragments out of the joint.

Sue, 36

"I've played volleyball really seriously since high school, in college, and then in various women's leagues. I began experiencing patellofemoral pain in my twenties, but it only got really bad in my early thirties. At first, it was just interfering with my ability to play as hard and as long as I would have liked, but by the time I went to a doctor, I was actually having difficulty walking.

I wasn't prepared to give up my sport, so when my doctor recommended an operation called a lateral release, I jumped at the opportunity for a "cure." Talk about unrealistic expectations. At the end of the day, not only wasn't it the miracle cure I had been expecting, but it didn't seem to do anything, to be perfectly honest, despite the fact that my surgeon pronounced it "successful" and I was really diligent about rehab. All that happened from my perspective was a missed season.

Now that I've been around the block a couple of times, I think that I should have investigated my non-surgical options a little more carefully.

What I really needed to do (and what has really worked for me since) is stretch. I've always been really strong and really inflexible—my husband used to tease me because, as athletic as I am, I'd never been able to touch my toes. And that whole band on the outside of my leg—my hip flexors, my iliotibial band—is always incredibly tight, and made worse because of my sport.

*I now do at least half an hour of stretching a day, four times a week. Once a month, I see my physical therapist, who stretches me out on a table, which not only feels amazing, but has made an incredible difference in my flexibility and range of motion. I not only touch my toes, but I'm back to playing full practices and games, without almost any pain under my kneecap at all (certainly nothing that an **Aleve** and some ice won't fix.)*

I realize that this isn't the only outcome from a lateral release—another woman on my team had one, and it was the "miracle cure" she needed (although she was good about physical therapy and stretching as well). I just feel like I did it backward, since I only learned about the importance of stretching after the surgery. If I'd known how important it was to work on flexibility on the outside of my leg, I would have liked to try that first, and I might not have needed surgery at all. "

How Long Will It Take to Recover?

Non-surgical. You can usually recover from patellofemoral syndrome with about six weeks of relative rest and rehabilitation, and orthotics, if appropriate. You should continue with your home stretching and strengthening programs after recovery. **You must correct whatever problems caused the condition, or you'll have a recurrence.**

Post-surgical. After a lateral release, you'll be on crutches for about a week, and then you'll need three to four months of physical therapy. Complete recovery can take up to six months.

Patella Fracture

Patellar fractures—the proverbial broken kneecaps—don't happen very often. A patellar contusion, or bruise, is more common and can be very painful. This can usually be treated with RICE.

The first thing to know about patellar fractures is there are different types—which affects the kind of symptoms you experience as well as your treatment options. If the fracture is undisplaced, the knee is left relatively intact. In a comminuted or stellated fracture, the bone has been splintered or crushed, creating a number of bone fragments. Single fractures are vertical, horizontal, and/or oblique (at an angle).

Men seem to get patellar fractures more than women do, which might have to do with their chosen activities. A patellar fracture may be caused by any number of things, but it's usually a force sustained directly on the kneecap, like falling down on your knees, or the kind of blow to the knee that's common in contact sports. They're a common injury in automobile accidents, from the kneecap smashing into the dashboard.

People with very weak bones—the elderly and the severely calcium deficient—may not need such dramatic forces to break their patellas. It's very common to see this condition in elderly women with osteoporosis, and sometimes the initiating injury was nothing more than banging the knee.

How Will I Know If I Have a Patellar Fracture?

You'll probably have acute pain around the kneecap. If something hit your patella, you might have heard the crack or pop of the bone breaking. The knee will probably swell immediately, you'll have quite a bit of pain, and movement will either be difficult or impossible. If pieces of the kneecap have actually separated from each other, your knee may appear to be deformed, and in some cases, you may actually be able to feel where the parts have separated.

When part of the broken bone pokes through the skin, it's called a **compound fracture**. These should also be treated as emergencies before you contract an infection.

You can also get a stress fracture of the patella, which we discuss in greater detail in the section on bone (pages 150-153).

How Will My Doctor Know
If I Have a Patellar Fracture?

Your doctor will examine your knee to test how difficult it is for you to extend your leg. The doctor will also see if it's possible to feel the different parts of the fracture. It's important that he check for intact quad and patellar tendons, since they are related to patella fractures. He will also look for swelling in the knee. Since the patella is a bone, your doctor will be able to use an X ray to determine whether or not the patella is fractured, and if so, what type of fracture it is. He may also order an MRI to see if there has been any related damage to the soft tissue.

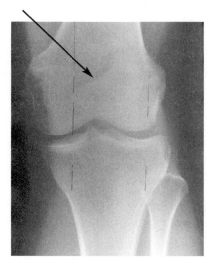

X-RAY OF PATELLA FRACTURE

> Note: about 1 percent of the population is born with an anatomical anomaly called **bipartite patella**, which simply means that the patella is made of two different bones not fused together, instead of a single bone. This condition is usually asymptomatic, but it can look like a fracture on an X ray.

WHAT ARE MY TREATMENT OPTIONS?

The way your patellar fracture is treated depends largely on the type of fracture it is. For nondisplaced fractures, your doctor will recommend a knee immobilizer for approximately four weeks, with weight bearing as tolerated.

Patellar reconstruction. If the damage has been more severe, an open-knee operation may be necessary to remove shards of bone from the knee and wire the existing fragments together, using wire, pins, or screws. Attention is paid to restoring the extensor mechanism—the way the quad, patella, and patellar tendon work together.

Patellar removal (patellectomy). In some very severe cases, total removal of the patella may be necessary. We tend to avoid doing this procedure because the patella plays such an important role in the extension of the knee, and removal of this bone does interfere with normal knee function. It can also interfere with the stability of a later knee reconstruction, since the muscles are no longer trained to support the kneecap.

Physical therapy. Surgery must always be followed by a program of physical therapy designed to restore proprioception, strength, and stability to the knee, like the General Knee Health Workout in Chapter 12 of this book.

HOW LONG WILL IT TAKE TO RECOVER?

Post-surgical recovery for a comminuted fracture takes about six to eight weeks—you're considered healed when an X ray shows that the bone has fused, although it may be another six months to a year of physical therapy before you're able to participate in activities at a preinjury level.

PATELLAR DISLOCATION OR SUBLUXATION

If the patella isn't tracking well in the trochlear groove, it can actually jump the track and become dislocated. This can be a really painful experience. If the patella jumps back into the groove after moving too far to the side, it's called *subluxation*, or partial dislocation.

HOW CAN I DISLOCATE MY PATELLA?

Sometimes dislocation is the result of a trauma. The most common cause of patellar dislocation is a mechanism very close to the one that causes most ACL injuries, which is why we see such a high incidence of these two injuries: a rotation of the knee while the foot is planted. So any sport that requires cutting, rapid changes of direction, or sudden stops, like basketball, tennis, and volleyball, puts you at higher risk for this condition.

Sometimes the problem is anatomical. People with large Q angles, miserable malalignment syndrome, people with knock-knees, or any internal rotation of the thighbone coupled with an external rotation of the shinbone may have less stability. Often, the trochlear groove is too shallow, or too shallow on one side, allowing the kneecap to more easily slip out of position. People who are inherently loose or double-jointed have a greater chance of subluxing or dislocating their patella, because the soft tissue restraints are generally much looser in these patients.

HOW WILL I KNOW IF MY PATELLA IS DISLOCATED?

If your kneecap is dislocated, you'll know. There will be great pain, usually accompanied by immediate swelling, and movement will be close to impossible. The knee will also look deformed, and you'll probably be able to see that the patella has been displaced.

A subluxation, or temporary dislocation, may be harder to see, because the kneecap will probably have replaced itself in the proper position, or close to it. You will have a feeling of instability and pain at the front of the knee, usually accompanied by swelling.

HOW WILL MY DOCTOR KNOW IF I'VE DISLOCATED MY PATELLA?

Your doctor will be able to tell if you have a dislocated patella with a physical exam. A patellar subluxation can be diagnosed through an examination of the kneecap itself, which may be loose in the track and feel tender and unstable to the touch.

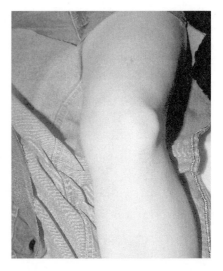

An X ray is not necessary to confirm the diagnosis but it may be helpful because it will tell your doctor if the dislocated patella ripped off a piece of the articular cartilage and bone, known as an **osteochondral fracture.**

DISLOCATED PATELLA

NON-SURGICAL TREATMENT OPTIONS

The treatment depends largely on the severity of the injury. When the patellofemoral ligaments have been severed, the treatment is immobilization.

RICE. Rest, ice, compression, and elevation, combined with NSAIDs, can help to alleviate the pain and speed healing of the subluxation. Avoid the activities that cause you pain. Icing after activity may help.

Bracing/taping. If your patella is prone to subluxation, your doctor may recommend that you brace or tape your patella before running, jumping, twisting, or cutting activities. Many patellar dislocations can be shifted back into place and immobilized by your doctor, much like a broken arm. You'll be in a splint for about four to six weeks.

Physical therapy. In the case of both subluxation and dislocation, a physical therapy program designed to strengthen the quadriceps muscles in the knee, especially the VMO is recommended. You'll find an appropriate Patellofemoral Health Workout in Chapter 12.

SURGICAL OPTIONS

Lateral release. In severe cases of repeated subluxation, your doctor may recommend an arthroscopic procedure called a lateral release. In this procedure, the lateral retinaculum, a structure on the outside of the leg, is partially cut, which relieves some of the pressure on the kneecap. Eventually, the ligaments that have been cut heal, and scar tissue fills in the gap left by the surgery. Sometimes the tendons on the inside of the leg need to be tightened as well.

Patellar realignment. In severe cases, a surgical procedure to change the place where the patellar tendon inserts on the tibia may be necessary, to change the forces on the patella.

Physical therapy. Surgery must always be followed by a program of physical therapy designed to restore proprioception, strength, and stability to the knee.

HOW LONG WILL IT TAKE TO RECOVER?

You'll be back on your feet at a light activity level about six to eight weeks after a subluxation, dislocation, or arthroscopy. Complete rehabilitation will take longer, up to six months. A more severe patellar dislocation can take up to a year to heal completely, especially if other parts of the knee were involved.

PLICA SYNDROME

The *plica* (plĭ-kah) is a band of tissue that makes a fold in the synovial lining; the word means "fold" in Latin. It's actually a remnant from our fetal development, part of the process of growing a knee in the first place. In some people, these vestigial folds never go away. Not everyone has them (about 50 to 60 percent of people do), and most people who do never even know that they're there.

But the plica can become thick and painful when it's irritated through overuse or injured through trauma. When the plica becomes thickened and inflamed, it can get pinched between the thighbone and the kneecap, interfering with the normal working of the joint. This is called plica syndrome. There are three major plicae, but plica syndrome is most commonly found in one of them: the *medial patellar plica*, on the upper inside of the knee. Women are more likely to experience plica syndrome than men are. See page 27 for an illustration of the plica.

HOW DOES PLICA SYNDROME DEVELOP?

There are two basic causes of plica syndrome. The first is trauma, such as a blow to the knee or a fall. I see a lot of these injuries after car accidents, for instance. The other is overuse. The plica can be irritated by repetitive stresses across the knee, especially ones that require the leg to be bent or straightened repeatedly. Bikers and long-distance runners sometimes have problems with their plica, and so do people who spend a lot of time on the Stairmaster at the gym. If you have anatomical irregularities or especially tight hamstrings, you're at higher risk.

HOW WILL I KNOW IF I HAVE PLICA SYNDROME?

Your symptoms may come and go. You may experience pain in the front or the inside of the knee joint, and swelling may occur. You'll probably feel tenderness over the area where the plica is, usually on the inside of the knee.

You may also hear something: a clicking, snapping or popping noise, as the plica snaps over one of the bumps on the bottom of the thighbone.

Thankfully, plica syndrome isn't usually associated with instability, but your knee may lock or feel weak. Anything that requires a lot of bending in the knee, such as deep knee bends or stairs, may be uncomfortable, and it may be worse when you sit for a long time, a condition known as theater knee.

HOW WILL MY DOCTOR KNOW IF I HAVE PLICA SYNDROME?

Your doctor will examine the knee to see where the pain is located. Sometimes, we can actually feel the swollen plica under the skin. Most of the time, a physical exam is sufficient for a diagnosis, but since plica syndrome shares many of the same symptoms of a meniscal tear, an MRI may be done to rule out the possibility of a tear. An X ray may also be ordered to make sure that there are no other bony problems in the knee. See page 27 for an illustration of the plica.

NON-SURGICAL TREATMENT OPTIONS

For the most part, plica syndrome can be treated conservatively.

RICE. Rest, ice, compression, and elevation, combined with NSAIDs, can help to alleviate the pain and speed healing. Ice may actually help your plica return to its normal size. Avoid the activities that cause you pain, especially anything that involves the repetitive bending and straightening of the knee.

Physical therapy. A program designed to strengthen the quadriceps and stretch the hamstring muscles in the knee without putting undue pressure on the patellofemoral joint is recommended. You'll find an appropriate Patellofemoral Health Workout program in Chapter 12 of this book.

Cortisone injections. If you're not having any luck with acetaminophen or the NSAIDs, corticosteroids are more powerful anti-inflammatory agents that can be injected directly into the plica or surrounding joint, reducing pain and swelling.

SURGICAL OPTIONS

If your case is severe and causing you a tremendous amount of pain, your doctor may recommend arthroscopic surgery to remove the irritating plica.

PART IV

GETTING BETTER

CHAPTER ELEVEN

PREPARING FOR SURGERY

When your injury has been properly diagnosed, you and your doctor will discuss your treatment options. If you've decided to take a more conservative approach, you can skip this chapter and go straight to the section on physical therapy. If you've decided that surgery is your best course of action, read this chapter first. You'll end up in physical therapy regardless!

The decision to undergo surgery, even a routine outpatient arthroscopy, is never a minor one and should not be undertaken lightly. You need to know how to find a surgeon and how to use your consultation with that surgeon to ensure that surgery is the best possible option for you. Once you've decided to go ahead with the procedure, there are any number of tips and tricks that I've picked up from my patients over the years that can help to make the experience—before, during, and after surgery—as seamless and trouble-free as possible.

It has been my experience that when patients feel they have participated in the decision to undergo surgery, they have a better prognosis.

They have a better attitude (and more realistic expectations) going into
the procedure. They're also more likely to get the rest they need, and
to commit to physical therapy over the long haul. So I think it's important for you to take a measure of control when you're contemplating
your options.

Surgery can be a scary and overwhelming process. Don't be intim-
idated: you have a right to know. You have a right to ask questions, and
to receive a full and satisfying explanation.

Here are some of the questions you may want to discuss with
your doctor:

— **Why is surgery my best option?** Make sure you've reviewed all
   of your available treatment options, and that you're satisfied with
   the decision the two of you have made. If you're not, get a second
   opinion. In fact, your health insurance may require that you get
   a second opinion before having certain types of surgery.

— **Why should I have surgery right now? What would happen if
   I delayed it?** Because there are so few instances where knee surgery
   is really an emergency, it's often worth talking about remedies,
   like Synvisc injections, that can "buy a little time." In most cases,
   deciding not to have surgery immediately doesn't mean that you
   can't have it eventually. Your doctor may present a compelling
   case for treatment sooner rather than later because certain injuries,
   like serious meniscal tears, can get worse over time, but it's a question that should be asked.

— **Is there something you can give me or recommend to read in
   order to learn more about the procedure?** Many of my patients
   express an interest in learning more about the procedure and
   the medical evidence for it. One of my patients, an art historian,
   jokes that she got an associate's degree in orthopedic surgery the
   summer before her total knee replacement. She simply felt more
   comfortable when she knew what she was heading into, and I
   was happy to give her the tools to do it. Your doctor may have
   a wide range of materials, from user-friendly patient information

handouts to more sophisticated medical journal articles to educational videotapes.

— **What are the chances of a full recovery?** "Recovery" is a variable term. It can depend on what kind of activity level you hope to return to, and will also be largely dependent on the amount of effort you yourself put into the rehabilitation process. Talk to your doctor about the factors in your particular case, the natural history of the procedure, and his or her expectations for you in particular.

— **What is a realistic expectation for the time it will take me to recover?** Although I've provided guidelines for many surgical procedures, your doctor will be able to tell you what a realistic recovery expectation is for you with a much greater degree of accuracy. That doesn't just mean a return to sports—there are lots of little milestones along the way. Find out when you can return to daily activities and work; when you'll be allowed to bear weight unassisted; when you'll be able to drive again; when you'll be able to return to your sport or activity.

— **What exactly will take place during the procedure? How long will the surgery take?** Your doctor should be able to explain the procedure in clear, layman's language, using visual aids if necessary. This is also a good time to find out whether or not there are different ways of doing the surgery. For instance, an anterior cruciate ligament (ACL) can be reconstructed using tendons from two different parts of the patient's leg, or donated tissue. If your surgeon is recommending one option over another, make sure you understand why that's the best strategy for you.

— **What are the risks?** Every surgical procedure has risks—for the joint that's being operated on, as well as for the patient's health at large. It's your doctor's responsibility to make sure that you're completely aware of the risks involved. At the same time, don't let yourself get too nervous about it—almost all of the procedures described in this book are performed regularly, and with a good success rate.

— **How long will the results last?** Many of the surgical procedures performed on the knee have limited life spans. For instance, a total knee replacement only lasts as long as the artificial joint does, and in a younger, more active person, that may not be your whole life. Your surgeon will be able to give you a ballpark estimate, based on his or her experience with the procedure, your age, and your activity level.

— **Will I need to have a blood transfusion? If so, is it possible to store my own blood in anticipation of the transfusion?** Many people feel more comfortable if they know their own blood will be used during the operation (if, in fact, any is needed at all). You'll want to find out if this is a possibility, and how you can make it happen if it is.

— **How much pain will there be? And how will my pain be managed before, during, and after the procedure?** There are three different kinds of anesthesia: local, which numbs a specific area, like a shot of novocaine at the dentist; regional, which numbs a part of the body, like the epidural that many women get during childbirth; and general, where you're knocked out completely. Your surgeon will be able to tell you what kind of anesthesia is appropriate for the procedure you're having, and any precautions that you should take in advance as a result. If you're planning to stay on pain medication before the surgery, you should discuss which medications he recommends since some increase bleeding and aren't advisable when you're going into surgery. You'll also want to have a conversation about the pain medication used immediately after the procedure, and the prescription you'll be sent home with.

— **How long will I have to stay in the hospital? Can this procedure be done on an outpatient basis?** Most of the arthroscopic surgeries described in this book can be done on an outpatient basis. More major surgeries will require a hospital stay. I find that people get better quicker if they're able to get home and into their own environment.

— **How long will I be confined to bed?** Depending on the nature of the surgery, your leg may be immobilized, but even if this is the case, you probably won't be confined to bed. We generally encourage patients to start moving around as soon as the day after the surgery.

— **When does my physical therapy start? How long will I need physical therapy? Can you recommend a facility?** Again, the answer will probably be "right away." The day of, or the day after your procedure, you'll almost certainly see a physical therapist who will start to encourage range of motion in your knee and who will be able to teach you some of the basic skills you'll need over the next few weeks, like how to get in and out of bed, use the bathroom, and use crutches.

— **How often will I see the doctor after the surgery, and when?** This answer depends on the procedure you've had done and your doctor's office policy. Your stitches will come out one to two weeks after the procedure. At four to six weeks, your doctor will want to examine your progress and discuss which activities you can resume. Expect to see your doctor a number of times after that to monitor your recovery until the injury is fully healed.

— **Should I discontinue any of the medications I'm taking in anticipation of surgery?** Make sure your surgeon knows which medications you take regularly—and don't leave anything out. For example, aspirin, a common NSAID and a staple item in most medicine cabinets, is a blood thinner and can cause excessive bleeding during surgery. Your surgeon may ask you to start taking acetaminophen (*Tylenol*) instead in the two weeks prior to the surgery.

When you're satisfied with the answer to these questions (and your own), you're ready to schedule the procedure. Sometimes, with a busy surgeon and a busy hospital, there may be a lag time, so there's no instant gratification there either. Use the time you have to prepare yourself well, and the procedure and its aftermath will go much better.

The Month Before

Learn as much as you can about the procedure. Continue to research the surgery on the Internet, and in books such as this one. You may also want to talk to someone else who's had the procedure. If you don't know anyone who's had it, ask your doctor. Sometimes when someone's feeling anxious about surgery, I'll connect them with another patient who's had the same operation. Hearing a non-medical person talk about the procedure—their own apprehension, their experience, and their recovery—can make an enormous difference in your attitude going into surgery.

REALISTIC EXPECTATIONS

I'm not going to sugar-coat this: knee surgery isn't a quick fix. Even if the procedure is minor, you will not be wheeled out of the operating room and onto the basketball court. Recovery requires time and a commitment to rehabilitation. If you have realistic expectations going into the procedure, and maintain them throughout your rehabilitation, you will be much less frustrated after the surgery is done.

Stay in shape. The wrong time to get lazy about your conditioning is when you're approaching surgery. The better the shape you're in when you go into the operating room, the better your chances of a complication-free procedure and a speedy recovery. If you're going to be off the leg for a while, you'll want to concentrate on your upper-body strength. Using crutches for any period of time takes a fair amount of strength.

Talk to your insurance company. Find out what's covered—and what isn't. How many nights of your hospital stay are covered? Is in-hospital rehab covered? Is temporary home care available? Do they cover follow-up visits with your surgeon, and how many of them?

Make sure you're not going to be ambushed by hidden costs. If you'll need physical therapy, a special brace, or a continuous passive motion machine, make sure these things are covered, and that they don't require preauthorization.

The Week Before

The week before the surgery, your doctor may ask you to go to the hospital for some routine tests, including X rays, as well as to give blood and urine samples. Other than that, you're on your own. Here are some of the ways you can use this time productively to prepare for the procedure.

TAKE CARE OF YOURSELF

If you smoke, stop. Nicotine can cause complications during and after surgery. Plus, the smoke-free zone of the hospital is a terrific place to kick-start your quitting effort!

Eat a balanced diet. The better nourished you are, the stronger your body will be. Ask your doctor if you should consider an iron supplement.

Drink plenty of fluids. The better hydrated you are, the faster you'll heal.

Rest.

If you have a cold, fever, respiratory infection, or any other infection, including any in your gums the week before surgery, let your doctor know.

SET UP YOUR HOUSE

— Make sure your house is well set up to accommodate you after the operation:

— Throw rugs and crutches don't mix. Roll them up and store them. Clear the floor space of anything that you can imagine getting in your way, and tape electrical cords to the floor or to the wall so that you don't trip.

— Leave clean laundry where it'll be easily accessible.

— Figure out how you're going to get in and out of the bath and on and off the toilet. You may need to install a bar to help you, or invest in an elevated toilet seat.

CALL THE HOSPITAL

If you're going to be staying in the hospital, you'll want to have some basic questions answered before you go in:

— If having a private room is important to you, if you require kosher or vegetarian food, or have other special needs that you'd like accommodated, find out whom you need to inform and when the appropriate time to do that is.

— Will there be a phone in your room? If not, is there a public phone on the floor? (Cellular phones are prohibited in hospitals, so you'll want to show up with plenty of quarters or a calling card if there's no phone in your room, or if you want to make a long-distance call.)

— Find out when visiting hours are, so that you can tell friends and family before the procedure.

STOCK UP ON SUPPLIES

— Grocery shop for staple items. Make and freeze batches of some of your favorite foods before the surgery so you can just pop a plastic container into the microwave in the early weeks of recovery.

— Following some surgeries, you won't be able to get your leg completely wet. Enter the Hefty bag! Use duct tape to secure a garbage bag around your leg, so make sure you have ample quantities of bags and tape stashed in the bathroom. Waterproof covers are also available from surgical supply houses.

— Shower seats are very useful, but the ones in surgical supply stores can be expensive. Any plastic chair with decent traction on the bottom will work—even an inexpensive lawn chair.

— You're not going to be going out on the town for a little while. Buy books and magazines, puzzles, and borrow some DVDs for your recovery.

— If you're going to need any other special items before surgery, this is a good time to pick them up.

ENLIST OR HIRE A CAREGIVER

— After the surgery, you will need help. How much help you need, and for how long, will depend on the severity of the procedure and your physical condition. Your doctor's office will be able to help you determine a realistic estimate.

— Arrange to have someone accompany you home from the hospital.

— Make sure you've made adequate child- and pet-care plans. Will it be a problem if you need to stay in the hospital an extra night or two?

— If no friend or relative can stay with you following surgery, talk to your doctor about the possibility of an extended-care facility or part-time in-home help.

INTERVIEW PHYSICAL THERAPISTS

This is a good time to start interviewing physical therapists and taking tours of the facilities they use. In the next chapter, I'll give you some tips on what to look for.

The Night Before

— Remove polish from your toenails and fingernails.

— Prepare to leave jewelry and other valuables at home. (Your wedding ring can be taped if it won't come off your finger.)

— Don't have anything to eat past 10 p.m., or anything to drink past midnight—not even water!—unless your surgeon or anesthesiologist has told you differently. No breath mints, or chewing gum either.

— Get plenty of sleep.

The Day of the Surgery

— Shower.

— Wear loose-fitting, comfortable clothing—and remember that you may be coming home with a brace, so figure that into your wardrobe decisions.

— Don't wear your contact lenses or your false teeth.

— If you'll need any medication, like insulin or an inhaler, bring them with you.

Before You Leave the Hospital

— Make sure a nurse or physical therapist has shown you how to use crutches.

— You should also be comfortable getting in and out of bed, and using the toilet.

— If you're in pain, make sure you have a prescription for medication, or have discussed alternative strategies with your doctor.

Crutches 101

After some knee surgeries, you'll be unable to bear weight on the involved leg, so you may be using crutches for a period of up to six or eight weeks. Unless you were an accident-prone kid, this may be your first time using these, and they're harder to use than they look. You probably don't want to be thinking about this for the first time in the hospital physical therapy room while you're on heavy-duty pain medication and dressed in a backless gown. So here are some pointers in advance:

— Keep your weight on your arms and hands, not on your armpits.

— Bend your elbows.

— Bend the involved knee, so that it doesn't skim the ground.

— Move both crutches forward, and swing your uninvolved leg between the crutches.

— Never use your crutches when you're going down stairs. Put them both under one arm and use the railing to support you as you hop down the stairs.

— In preparation for surgery, you'll want to build as much upper-body strength as possible. The stronger you are, the easier it'll be for you to use your crutches for extended periods of time, and the less trapped and immobile you'll feel after the surgery.

— A patient shared the following crutch survival secret: the fanny pack. This is a small bag that you tie around your waist, and it functions as a big pocket—an invaluable aid when you're moving around your house on crutches, and don't have the use of your hands.

In the Immediate Recovery Period (The Week After Surgery)

— Try to move around as much as possible, increasing your activity level as you feel you can. Don't stay in bed!

— If you've been sent home with some light physical therapy exercises before your first official physical therapy appointment, do them diligently.

— You'll likely be flooded with well-wishers. Put them to work! When a friend asks "What can I do to help?" give them specific instructions. Ask them if they'd mind picking up groceries, or pet food, or refilling your prescription for you. Before they arrive, make a small list of the tasks around the house that you can't do for yourself (something incredibly minor like reaching something on a high shelf or bending down to get something can be incredibly frustrating and painful immediately after knee surgery), and ask them to run and fetch for five minutes before they leave.

— Keep the wound clean and dry until your doctor says it can get wet.

When Should I Call My Surgeon?

Following surgery, how will you know what are real warning signs that you should pay attention to, and what is normal?

Call your surgeon if:

— you're having difficulty breathing.

— your calf or foot is painful, swollen, or red—or if there's no feeling there at all.

— the wound seems to be infected—i.e., if it's red and hot to the touch.

— you have a fever of over 101 degrees.

■ CHAPTER TWELVE ■

PHYSICAL THERAPY

Whether part of your post-surgical recovery, or used in lieu of surgery, physical therapy is a crucial part of recuperating from an injury or chronic condition, and can dramatically affect the future stability and strength of the knee.

What Does a Physical Therapist Do?

Physical therapists are there to guide you as you relieve pain, restore function to your knee, and improve your mobility. They tend to have a strong educational background in subjects like anatomy, biology, physiology, biomechanics, exercise physiology, and neuroanatomy, and they're trained to evaluate and treat knee pain in coordination with your treating physician.

While you're in therapy, your physical therapist is your knee's advocate. He will push you to do the best thing for your knee—even when you don't want to. He'll help you to protect the knee from irritating actions before they occur. And he'll teach you how to take care of your-self, developing healthy knee habits that you can take with you even after you leave therapy.

How Do I Find a Therapist?

Your doctor will probably have a physical therapist or physical therapy group he works with. If you're comfortable with that person and the facility, it's probably worth it to go there. It's important for your doctor to have a good working relationship with your physical therapist. In my experience, the team approach works best. Your doctor may come up with protocols and guidelines regarding healing constraints ("don't move it past 90 degrees for six weeks," or "no weight bearing for three weeks"), but it's the therapist's job to develop and implement these and to continue to access the patient during the rehab process so they can partner with the physician to tweak that protocol to accommodate the patient's changing needs.

If that doesn't work out, go back to word of mouth. If you know anyone—or know anyone who knows anyone!—who's been through physical therapy, and had a good experience with the therapist and the facility, that's your next best route. If you've had surgery, and liked the person you saw at the hospital, you might call to inquire about their availability, or to find out if they can recommend a colleague.

You can also contact:

The American Physical Therapy Association (APTA)
1111 North Fairfax Street
Alexandria, VA 22314-1488
Phone: 800 999-APTA (2782)
TDD: 703 683-6748
Fax: 703 684-7343
Fax on Demand: 800 399-APTA (2782)
www.apta.org

APTA members are held to a rigorous code of ethics and behavior. They keep a database of licensed member physical therapists (searchable on their website), and will be happy to help you find one in your area. All physical therapists have to be licensed to practice in their state; some states even require continuing education to maintain a license.

Again, if at all possible, do use the physical therapist recommended by your physician.

What I Should Look For in a Physical Therapist and Treatment Facility?

Your specifications for a physical therapist are similar to the ones you should have for finding a doctor. In this case, though, a personal relationship really is important. A physical therapist should be someone with whom you feel comfortable talking and asking questions. You're going to be spending a lot of time together, and you need to feel that this person can help you to get better.

Your sports medicine physician will refer you to a physical therapist who specializes in sports medicine and musculoskeletal injuries. If you find your physical therapist in any other way, it's important to establish their level of experience in this area. Physical therapy is a broad field, and while what the education therapists receive is broad, most of them specialize once they leave school. Someone might be terrific with head injuries, but that won't help your knee.

If you find a physical therapist who's also certified as an athletic trainer and/or a fitness professional, that's excellent. An athletic trainer is the person on the sidelines at a sporting event who runs onto the field when someone gets injured. Since they work with sports-related injuries exclusively, they have real expertise and hands-on knowledge. It's certainly not a requirement, but it will mean that the therapist has a significant sports medicine background, and that training generally translates into an approach that emphasizes keeping active people active. You'll find that many physical therapists are now training under the supervision of athletic trainers, gathering experience on the sidelines.

When you call the facility, ask how much one-on-one time you'll get with the physical therapist himself (as opposed to an assistant). The closer the answer is to half an hour, the better. (If you can afford it, even periodically, it's really worth it to work one-on-one with a therapist.) The facility itself should be clean and well-equipped, with private treatment rooms and open mat space for functional exercises and stretching.

You should see people getting a fair amount of individual attention; you don't need to be baby-sat while you're on the elliptical trainer or the stationery bike, but you should have the feeling that people are being attended to and that they're getting face time with a therapist, not just a legion of assistants. And you should see people doing different things for different injuries.

The Right Attitude—Yours!

No discussion of physical therapy would be complete without a reminder about how very important your own attitude and full participation is in your recovery. "You get out what you put in to it" is true in general about physical performance—people in great shape are generally that way because they educate themselves and then log the hours, doing the work. This is never more true than when you're recovering from an injury.

No matter how good your physical therapist is, he can't make you better—only you can make you better. You have to fully commit to the time and energy this is going to take. PT is hard work. It can be tiring. Sometimes it hurts. Sometimes it's not convenient. You may get to a point and think: "That's it—I'm done. I can live with a knee that isn't perfect." But when you cheat at your physical therapy, you just cheat yourself.

If you feel yourself starting to flag, don't give in and quit. Do something. Keep a journal. Join one of the knee injury websites with a community forum, so you can share your frustrations and triumphs with other people in a similar position. Keep an inspirational quote above your desk. Talk to a friend. Tell your physical therapist that you're starting to get overwhelmed, and see how he responds. This might be a good time to splurge on a one-on-one session with him, just to get you out of the rut you're in. Call your doctor if you feel you're not progressing.

The better your attitude is toward this process, the better your knee will recover. When you do make and stick to that commitment, you'll be richly rewarded—not only by the way your knee functions now, but by the bullets you're ducking in the future as well.

How Will I Know If It's Working?

Sometimes progress in physical therapy feels incredibly slow. But you will notice a difference. The first thing you'll notice may be a change in the amount and intensity of pain you feel. For instance, you may feel pain all day, but not as intensely as you did before. Or the pain may be just as intense, but only after a long day of activity, instead of all the time. As you continue with the therapy, the pain will continue to abate, and you should notice that your symptoms change: you have increased range of motion and strength, your activities of daily living become easier, and your leg begins to look more conditioned and healthy.

If you feel you've diligently put in the time and you still aren't seeing results, it's something to discuss with your therapist and your doctor— and may be a reason to find another therapist.

Your First Session

In your first meeting, your physical therapist will take your personal medical history and the history of the injury or pain.

He'll test your strength by having you push against him with both your injured and noninjured legs: you may have suffered a certain amount of atrophy in your muscles, and he may measure around both to determine how much wasting has occurred in the injured leg or how much swelling is present. He'll also ascertain where you are in terms of flexibility, range of motion, balance, and coordination. He'll ask you about the level and location of pain you currently feel. He'll take notes on your general fitness condition, including your natural alignment, posture, cardiovascular performance, and muscle tone. If you've had surgery, he may check the incision and talk to you about wound care. He'll talk to you about your goals, and the level of activity you'd like to return to.

Then, and only then, will he start to talk to you about a possible treatment strategy. At the end of this meeting, ask your new physical therapist for a treatment plan: your mutual goals, eventual prognosis, how long he expects it will take, and what it will take to get there.

Jennifer, 30

"It's strange to hear someone say that their knee injury ended up being the best thing that ever happened to them, but in my case, it just might be true. I was twenty-two when I ruptured my ACL. I'd like to be able to tell a glamorous story about the way I injured myself, but in fact I was replacing a book on a bookshelf in my office and swiveled to answer the phone. I heard the classic pop and went down hard. The pain was blinding, and I could tell right away that something serious had happened.

I wasn't comfortable with the first doctor I went to, although he came highly recommended and had a lot of celebrity clients. I felt rushed in his office, and when I expressed anxiety about the idea of surgery, I felt that he was dismissive of my concerns. I ended up going to an orthopedic surgeon recommended by my boss's wife, who'd fractured her elbow a couple of years before. He also felt that surgery was the best route, mostly because I was so young. So we scheduled an ACL repair, using my hamstring tendon.

The surgery went well, and so did my recovery. I walked without support in a couple of weeks, and started physical therapy—and here's where the good part starts. It sounds ridiculous, but I loved physical therapy! Now, I'd struggled with my weight my whole life, and hated anything that looked remotely like exercise. But I had a terrific physical therapist, and there was something about seeing appreciable gains in my injured leg that really appealed to me. My knee became my new project, and I was going to do anything and everything I could to get it back in great working shape. And as I was rehabilitating my knee, I was learning about the way my body worked—how to do exercises properly, the importance of proper technique, how muscle groups work together, and the most effective ways to strengthen them. I'd never thought of my body as a system before, just parts.

I paid out-of-pocket to continue PT, and when I could no longer do that, I joined an inexpensive gym and did my workouts there. Once my healing was more or less complete, I started to experiment with other exercises outside of my protocol. I had already started to build other parts of my body, not just the muscles I needed to support my knee, and I was starting to see real visible gains there as well. In other words, I discovered exercise, and I ended up getting into—and staying in—good shape.

I now work out at the gym three times a week, doing a combination of cardio and weights. I do Pilates two or three times a week as well, and just went to my first yoga class. I'll never be a size four, but for the first time in my life, I'm not self-conscious about my body; I feel strong and healthy, because I look strong and healthy. I know I never would have made the discovery on my own, and I think my ACL scar is a small price to pay!"

The Stages of Rehabilitation

As with any recovery process, there are stages to physical rehabilitation. In the very first days, sometimes the goal is just to decrease pain, reintroduce movement, protect the joint, and increase your range of motion a few degrees. The intermediate stage is about rebuilding. And the final stage is the essential fine polish: sports- or life-specific training that will allow you to return to your previous level of activity.

Obviously, your starting point depends on the degree of injury you've sustained. Someone who's had a light arthroscopic surgery is going to have a head start on someone who's just had three ligaments reconstructed or a complete joint replacement. And, of course, these stages overlap. There's no line in the sand when you cross from stage two to stage three: some of the things you do on the first day of stage one ultimately affect how rapidly and well stage three will go. You might achieve some goals rapidly, and others slowly. So I'd encourage you to think of these stages as part of a continuum, not as clearly demarcated boxes. This is why none of them can be skipped, and why it's impossible to assign an amount of time to each one.

> **Note:** Every physical therapist works differently, using some or all of the modalities described in this chapter. If something sounds interesting to you, you might want to inquire about it.

The First Stage: Getting You Back on Your Feet

Whether or not you've had surgery, after an injury the first stage is to get you back on your feet. You may need help using your assistive devices, like crutches, or to be fitted with a brace, and a physical therapist can help you with those things.

The more swollen you are, the harder it is to move, which makes it harder to regain range of motion, so getting some of that early post-trauma swelling down is the first order of business. This will probably involve a combination of ice, compression, and massage. If you had surgery, your doctor may also have prescribed a *continuous passive motion* (CPM) machine, that moves your leg back and forth for you. It can help to redistribute fluid and reduce swelling (especially when used in combination with cold therapy), keep the joint active to prevent scarring, and increase range of motion.

In a few weeks, you will need to be weaned off crutches, to bear weight unassisted on your leg and to learn to walk heel-to-toe again. This is harder than it sounds: if you haven't been able to bear weight on your involved leg, then you may be surprised at the amount of reluctance you feel when it comes time to shift your weight to the leg on the side that hurts. Your physical therapist will help you as you practice walking, monitoring your steps to make sure that they're equal in length so you don't recover with a limp, and will make sure that you can negotiate stairs unassisted.

I don't advise patients to self-medicate with heat, because ice is usually preferred except in specific circumstances, but a physical therapist will know when the joint needs better circulation and has the tools, like an ultrasound machine, which uses high-frequency waves to generate heat to implement this therapy in a way that causes no damage.

There's also a technology called *functional electrical stimulation* (FES), which can help your muscle regenerate itself, and relieve pain and swelling. Flat pads containing electrodes are placed over the muscle, and a light electrical current is passed through the skin, stimulating the nerves. This causes a muscle contraction, without any effort on your part. Eventually, as you regain control of the muscle, you can begin to tighten it yourself when you feel the electricity begin.

You need to begin to regain your range of motion so the structures in the knee don't get bound by scar tissue. There are a number of ways your physical therapist can help you to achieve this: active range of motion (when you do a stretch or a range of motion exercise by yourself); passive range of motion (when the therapist does it for you); active assisted (you do what you can, and the therapist helps). Your physical therapist may also use massage, specifically soft tissue manipulation, to break up scar tissue and increase the range of motion in the joint.

The next step is to awaken the other muscles in your leg. For instance, your therapist may encourage you to flex and point your foot, or to start rebuilding the quadriceps muscles, using a static contraction and release technique. This will help to reduce the swelling and help you regain strength. When you can bend your knee 70 degrees, you can start to work on a stationary bicycle.

Once you've achieved a fuller range of motion and the swelling has been significantly reduced, you're ready to begin a more active stretching and strengthening program.

The Second Stage: Rebuilding

The next stage of your therapy is to rebuild the machine: you have to increase your strength, regain your balance, continue to maximize your range of motion and flexibility, and continue to rebuild your endurance. This can be a slow process, but it's less frustrating if you realize how many components there are, and how much you're actually *doing*.

Let's take a closer look at what that all really means, and how your physical therapist will help you do it.

Build your core strength. After an injury or a surgery, you need to build strength. That's a given. But that doesn't simply mean a narrow-minded focus on the quads and the hamstrings, the muscles that cross the knee directly. You'll also need to concentrate on the muscles that support the knee, like the buttocks, hips, pelvis, abs, and back. Having strong legs is only half the battle; these core muscles are directly linked to the knee and provide the foundation for the body's overall balance and strength. If your core is weak, your body will be weak, so any rehabilitative effort must also include core strength. It's easy to get tunnel vision about your legs, especially when you're training for a sport or rehabilitating an injury. I believe that our general lack of focus on core strength is one of the reasons we're in such a knee crisis.

Physical therapists have a saying: "Proximal stability for distal mobility." Proximal means close to the body; distal means away from it. To translate: a strong foundation at the core means greater control over and better performance in the extremities.

Much of core strength training is an effort to develop a balance between the anterior and the posterior musculature—a balance between the abs and the lower back, the front of the pelvis and the buttocks. We do have a tendency to work on what we see in the mirror and to neglect what we cannot. It's no surprise, then, that the weaker structures at the back of the body, like the hamstrings, the rotator cuff, and our lower backs are the ones that get injured, or cause injuries elsewhere in the body.

Build your functional strength. Functional exercises are designed to mimic the activities that we all perform over the course of an average day. After all, what's sitting down in a chair if not a form of a squat? The beauty of functional exercises are that they make all those real activities, like sitting down in a chair (or the bucket seats in a sports car) much easier.

The key to the functionality of many of these exercises—and to their ease on your joints—is that they work on what we call a closed kinetic chain, which means that they're done with your feet against something solid, like the ground.

The other key with these exercises: like the functional activities they replicate, they involve multiple joints and muscle groups working together. So you're often getting a core body workout and building your balance at the same time that you're reinforcing your quadriceps muscles. This speeds the progress you'll see.

Build your eccentric strength. As part of this concept of balance, it's important to understand that there are two different kinds of strength: concentric and eccentric. The concentric is the "positive" part of the movement—flexing your elbow in a biceps curl, for instance, is concentric. The "negative" part of a movement, the lowering of the weight, is the eccentric movement. During the eccentric contraction, the muscle is forced to lengthen to decelerate the body. Eccentric movements are harder on the body. Unfortunately, they're also often neglected, which can result in injury.

JUMPING

As we've seen over the course of this book, many knee injuries happen while an athlete is jumping. Why is this particular activity such a hazard?

Jumping happens to be an action that combines both eccentric and concentric movements. You preset your joints before you jump by going into a slight squat. This is an eccentric movement. Then you explode upward into the jump itself, a concentric movement. As you land, you go back into a squat, another eccentric movement. A large component—the beginning and the end—of that movement is an eccentric load. If you don't train eccentrically so your body is equipped to handle that load, you're prone to injury in the first and last phases of the movement.

Get back in balance. As you know by now, muscle strength is crucial, but it certainly isn't the only thing lost when you have an injury, and it's only one contributor to knee injury prevention. Another biggie is balance—that all-important concept that I keep returning to in this book.

I mean balance in the literal sense (being able to stand on one leg, for example) and I'll talk about that a little later, but also balance in the body. For instance, it's absolutely essential that the inside of your leg be as conditioned as the outside. It can never be as strong as the outside, because it's not as big, but when it's well conditioned, there are no discrepancies in the amount of time it takes your brain to send a message to both muscle groups and the time it takes them to respond. Something similar is true about the front and the back of the body. The muscles at the back of the body are probably never going to be as strong as those in the front (in fact, an acceptable quad/hamstring ratio is around 3:2), but you can work toward that ideal, and if your hamstrings are as well conditioned as your quads, then you're at reduced risk for injury. This kind of balance takes a conscious effort on our part, and as a result, it's true of very few of us.

Any number of problems present themselves when your body is out of balance. You'll always have a tendency to rely more heavily on the stronger muscles, which forces the body out of its normal mechanics and puts undue strain on the knees. A classic example of this is the difficulty we see with female athletes, because they are often much stronger in the front of their bodies than they are at the back. This makes them fast out of the gate, but when they come down from a jump, an activity that demands that they engage the decelerator muscles, they don't have the strength or flexibility to sustain the move, and they end up with injuries.

There's a general rule with the body: unless you step in and change the dynamic, what is strong will stay strong, and what is weak will get weaker. Nowhere is this more true than after an injury. When you're hurt, your body automatically compensates to protect the structure that's hurt by doing double-duty with one that isn't. And the resulting imbalance can have disastrous results.

This question of timing is one that we'll continue to explore. Often, it's not a lack of strength that causes knee injury as much as a lack of conditioning that results in poor timing. Ideally, when your brain sends a message to your leg, you want all the muscles recruited at the same time. But if one side is significantly better conditioned, then that side is going to respond first. Take biker's knee, or anterior knee pain, as an example. This often results from the patella getting dragged to one side of the track it glides in, instead of in the center. Every time you push down on your pedals, the two sides of your knee are battling for control of your patella. Because the outside of your leg is stronger and better conditioned, it tends to be faster, and it wins the skirmish, dragging your patella off to the side. Do that a few hundred thousand times, and you're going to have a very irritated knee. This is a problem that's solved if the inside and the outside muscles of the leg are balanced and equally conditioned.

Physical balance, the amount of control you exercise over your center of gravity, is also important. The simplest tasks, like sitting down in a chair, require a modicum of balance and body awareness, and it's certainly a core competency for all of our sports and activities. When we're injured or weak, this is one of the first things to go, and one of the last to come back, so many of the exercises in our programs hone this skill even while they strengthen and stretch our muscles.

TEST YOUR QUAD TIMING

Sit up, with a flat back and your legs extended in front of you. Place a rolled towel underneath the knee you're working. Place three fingers of one hand on the muscle tissue above the shallow hollow on the inside of your kneecap. Place three fingers of the other hand on the middle of the outside of the leg. Quickly make a muscle by pushing the back of your knee into the pillow, *keeping the heel down and in contact with the floor.* Release the muscle.

Now close your eyes and remember what you felt through your hands. Did the inside and the outside of your leg fire at the same time, or was there some lag between them?

If you're like most people, chances are good that there was a little lag time. That's because most of us are better conditioned on one side of the body than on the other. So it's not so much a *strength* issue as one of *timing*—or timing as a result of decreased neuromuscular control. All that means is that the pathway between the brain and the nerve receptors in the muscle in your inner thigh are different from the pathway to your outer thigh, which is getting the message from the brain and reacting to it at a different time.

If you discovered that there was some lag time, you know that you have some work to do on the different muscles of your thigh to get it up to speed. This imbalance can cause injury over time, but strengthening the inner quadriceps muscle, for example, will significantly help to improve muscle recruitment time.

Know the Importance of Proprioception and Kinesthetic Awareness. Closely related to balance is the concept of **proprioception**, or the understanding of where your limb is in space at any given time. (When you're moving, this is called *kinesthetic awareness.*)

When you feel an itch, you're usually able, without error, to put your finger on the exact place that has the itch. That's proprioception. Your nerves and tiny receptors located all over your body sent your brain a message, and your brain followed the directions to the location of the itch. Kinesthetic awareness is essentially proprioception in motion: it's an understanding of where your limb is when it's *moving* through space. When you're walking, one foot is on the ground and one is swinging forward. The foot on the ground requires proprioception, and the one that's moving requires kinesthetic awareness.

Every time you do something simple like getting up off the couch and walking over to the refrigerator, you're using your proprioception and kinesthetic awareness. Your body is making hundreds of minute calculations, like how far you need to stretch out your arm to grab the door handle, and how far back you need to stand from the refrigerator so you don't hit your body when you open the door, all based on the information it receives from the specialized receptor cells in your various limbs. Athletes are using this information at an accelerated rate: when you're running down the sideline and make a quick cut to avoid an oncoming linebacker, your brain isn't asking, "Is my knee stable? How many degrees will I have to shift in order to successfully make this move?"—you just *do* it.

When you have surgery or an injury, those receptors cells are damaged, and the result is a loss of that "joint sense." It's not unusual to see post-surgical patients genuinely surprised at the places their legs have ended up in therapy. A normally well-coordinated person can become uncoordinated. The brain is sending messages, and the nerve receptor cells are sending messages back, but there's static over the lines. Now, these cells may be damaged, but we can easily recruit other cells from noninjured structures to make up for them, so that other cells are able to accurately describe the position of the limbs to the brain.

You may start with exercises as deceptively simple as standing on one leg or stepping up on a step to improve your kinesthetic awareness. Eventually, your therapist may ask you to use a balance board, similar to the ones that surfers train on, or even just to stand on one leg on an uneven surface or something soft like foam.

It is incredibly important to regain these skills. First of all, they are core competencies, so whether you're a pro athlete or a couch potato, you require them for everything they do. And unless you rebuild these skills along with your strength, you're at serious risk for re-injury. You're not ready to go back to full activity just because your bones have fused, or because you've regained your quad strength—these other important ingredients have to be in place as well. As you'll see in our workout programs in this chapter, closed kinetic chain exercises are also good at upgrading your balance, proprioception, and kinesthetic awareness. Because your foot is fixed, your knee has to be stable and secure to support your upper body.

Build Endurance. The muscles in our legs aren't the only ones that suffer when we get injured—our hearts and lungs get out of shape, too. An important part of physical therapy is to rehabilitate not only the joint but your cardiovascular system.

It's hard to do cardio with a serious knee injury, but it's not impossible. Your physical therapy facility probably has an upper-body ergometer, which is like a bike for your arms, and it's a great way to get your heart rate up. You can swim, using a foam buoy to keep your legs afloat while your arms do all the work. If your leg is healing well, you can use the stationary bike, which will help to strengthen the leg as well.

By the end of the second stage of rehab, you should basically be back to normal function.

COPING WITH PAIN

It's no secret: sometimes physical therapy hurts. But PT really doesn't stand for "pain and torture"—and if it feels as if it does, you may be overdoing it.

So how can you differentiate between "the good hurting," which happens when you necessarily push your leg a little farther with every session, crucial steps if you want to make progress, and "bad" hurting, which means that you're doing further damage to an already insulted joint? Here are some basic guidelines to help you gauge whether your pain is normal or something to worry about:

— Everyone is familiar with serious muscle soreness—the feeling you have after your first real day of skiing at the beginning of a season, the day after you've shoveled a heavy snowfall, or a day spent gardening. It hurts, sometimes a lot, but no matter how bad it gets, it's clearly soreness and not an injury. That's the good hurt. You may be sore the day after therapy (in fact, you probably will be), and you may be even sorer the day after (this is called delayed onset muscle soreness), but the soreness should have started to dissipate by the third day. In the meantime, you may take an NSAID and do some mild cardiovascular activity, like walking or gentle cycling.

— If, on the other hand, you have real pain at the joint line or underneath the kneecap, you need to tell your therapist, and he needs to adjust the exercises you're doing by reducing the weight or the range of motion you're using. The most important thing is for you to maintain good communication with your therapist. Talk to him about how long it hurts after therapy, and where. Describe the type of pain you feel. He'll tell you whether it's normal or not.

— The same thing goes with crepitus, or the crunching you hear in your knee. Some crunching may be normal, the same way your feet crack sometimes when you're walking barefoot. But really loud persistent crunching and cracking should be addressed when accompanied by pain, and may mean that you're doing the exercise wrong or too deeply for your own good. This is something else to discuss with your therapist and doctor.

— Pain, when your physical therapist is manipulating you, is also not uncommon. That's usually because he's pushing through scar tissue that's causing an adhesion in the joint. This is acceptable (although you should tell him you're feeling pain)—*but you should never feel any pain at all when you're self-treating.* A trained professional knows exactly what he's doing—which parts of the knee are involved, what's being compressed, and how much pressure is required to achieve his desired goal without incurring further injury. You don't. So leave it in his hands, and stop if you feel pain when you're working alone.

Third Stage: Fine-Tuning Your Recovery

The third stage of physical therapy continues to build on the foundation laid by the earlier ones. Often, this level is specific to the sport you'd like to return to—both enhancing your performance when you return and preventing a recurrence of the injury.

The balance, proprioception, and kinesthetic awareness exercises will get more sophisticated. Instead of standing on one leg for thirty seconds, you might stand on one leg with your eyes closed for a full minute, for instance. You'll also be working on regaining speed and power.

You may also begin some sport-specific exercises. A basketball player will learn how to jump and how to land with her knees bent and her hamstrings engaged, for instance. A soccer player might start to do footwork and agility drills. A martial artist might practice jumping up and landing on the same leg on an unstable surface. If the physical therapy is good and thorough enough, you may go back to your sport faster and more skilled than you were before you were injured. And these exercises perform another essential function: they're not only rehabilitative but preventive, and will make you considerably less prone to injury in the future.

You don't need to become an "expert" to avoid or overcome injury, but you may need to learn some new habits. If your injury was caused by problems in your training or correctible anatomical irregularities, your therapist can help you fix these problems so the injury doesn't recur. This is one of the physical therapist's most important roles.

Your physical therapist will also help you continue therapy on your own, with a home program of exercises designed to fit your needs. If you're going to continue working with a personal trainer or other fitness professional, it may be worth it for the two of them to meet and exchange notes, so your future training builds on, instead of compromising, your results.

Do I Really Need a Physical Therapist?

Many of my patients want to know if they can do their rehab on their own, and in many instances this is appropriate. At other times, especially with a more involved injury (or if you have self-discipline problems), I do recommend that you see a professional, if only for a couple of sessions. You'll go further in a shorter amount of time with a professional, and a physical therapist can assist in designing an at-home therapy program for you.

A physical therapist can:

Make sure you're doing the exercises properly. In the best case scenario, doing the right exercises the wrong way wastes your time. In the worst, it puts you at risk for serious re-injury—or doing new damage. Even subtle changes in exercise protocols can make a dramatic difference in the muscles affected and the stress placed on the joint. It's not hard to learn to do these correctly, but you have to learn. And, especially in the first sessions, your physical therapist can make sure that there are no major complications in the way your injury is healing.

Give you access to sophisticated treatment and rehab modalities. Your physical therapist probably has access to tools that can make rehab easier. You may be more comfortable exercising in a warm pool, for instance. Electrical stimulation may help your muscles recover faster. You certainly don't need to work out with a biofeedback unit, which tells you which muscles are working and how hard, but it can help. Some advanced exercises shouldn't be done except under supervision.

Monitor your progress. The leading cause of re-injury is when patients go and do things they're not ready to do. One of a physical therapist's most important functions is to know what you're ready for and what you're not. Don't second-guess him or push past the guidelines you've been given, even if you're feeling better and can perform movements without pain. If you do, you may end up taking a step backward in your rehab—or unwittingly set yourself up for future problems.

Keep you honest. Even the most disciplined person cheats every once in a while, and there are going to be days when you feel more like watching a *Seinfeld* rerun than doing that third set of leg presses. You may also have a tendency, even if you're keeping the remote safely out of sight, to "cheat" a little on the exercises that aren't as comfortable for you—in short, exactly the ones you need to be doing extras of! A physical therapist can protect you against yourself—and cheerlead when you need a little extra energy boost.

The following exercises were designed by a leading sports physical therapist and strength and conditioning professional, and will put much of what you've learned in this chapter into actual practice.

The Exercise Workouts

Whether you're rebuilding your strength after a major injury or surgery, working to increase your range of motion as part of your strategy to cope with arthritis, or strengthening and stretching the muscles to support the knee so you won't have to contend with the possibility of knee injury, there's something in the following exercises for you.

We've divided the exercises in this chapter into five separate workouts. If you're recovering from an injury or from surgery, you should consult with your physician and physical therapist before you use these workouts as rehab. They may want to alter the protocols to optimize the workout for you and your specific injury profile.

WHO SHOULD USE WHICH WORKOUT—AND HOW OFTEN?

The **Stretching Workout** stretches the muscles that support the knee, and is appropriate for everyone. Ideally, you'd stretch every day, but this workout should absolutely precede every one of the muscle strengthening workouts provided, and in fact, it's a good idea to do it before any kind of workout or physical activity. The **Core Strength Workout** targets abdominal and back muscles, and is an important component in preventing and rehabilitating knee pain and injury. You should do this workout about two times a week.

Our **General Knee Health Workout** is a preventive program designed to build and strengthen the knee's stabilizing muscles so that the joint is less vulnerable to injury and pain. You should do this workout three times a week. The **ACL Health Workout** is for people recovering from a stretched or torn ACL—and for anyone at high risk for ACL injury who wishes to strengthen the muscles that support this crucial ligament. The **Patellofemoral Health Workout** is designed for those who have experienced patellofemoral pain and/or meniscal injury. These strengthening workouts should be done three to five times a week, preferably on alternate days.

Each of these workouts should take about 30 to 45 minutes to complete. For those days when it's not possible to dedicate this time to your knee, we've included the "On the Run" Stretching and Strength Workout, a combination of three essential stretches and three essential strengthening exercises to do when you're pinched for time.

GENERAL NOTES ON THE WORKOUTS

— Remember, you should consult with a doctor before beginning any exercise program. Exercise does put additional strain on the heart, and you don't want to unwittingly put yourself in danger. Although these exercises should be safe no matter what kind of injury you had, your sports medicine physician, physical therapist, or fitness professional may want to make modifications to maximize the benefits you receive.

— Try not to rest more than one or two minutes between sets. That way, you'll get some cardiovascular benefits as well.

— You may not be able to complete the workout as given immediately. Gradually work up to the number of sets and repetitions given below.

— Perform these strengthening exercises three to five times per week, preferably on alternate days. Take a day off if you experience a great deal of soreness.

— All of these exercises should be done PAIN-FREE. If you're using weights and feeling pain, first decrease the range of motion. If you're still feeling pain, drop back on the weight and increase the range of motion to normal. If pain persists, drop back on both the weight and the range of motion. If there's no weight involved, simply decrease the range of motion. If pain continues after you've done all these things, discontinue the exercise, and try again when you're a little stronger.

— As you get stronger and more fit, these exercises will present less of a challenge. You can always increase their intensity by 1) holding the exercise a little longer; 2) increasing the number of repetitions you do; 3) adding a set; 4) adding weight or resistance, such as placing an ankle weight above the knee or at the ankle, or by adding weight to the fitness machine indicated. We've included "Challenge Yourself!" suggestions of ways that you can modify the exercises to increase the amount of difficulty they present.

THE STRETCHING WORKOUT

As we've seen, many serious knee injuries can be the result of overly tight muscle structures around the knee. The body's natural defense against stress, whether that stress is physical or emotional, is to tighten up the muscles. So stretching encourages the body to let go of that stress.

Stretching will also improve your sports performance. For instance, loosening a runner's tight hamstrings can automatically lengthen their stride and lead to improved running times.

You should stretch at the beginning and the end of your workout. If it's a rest day, you should stretch anyway! Plus, it will help with soreness.

Do not, under any circumstances, bounce while you're stretching. This is called ballistic stretching and can cause serious damage to the muscles.

I generally recommend that you hold stretches for a minimum of 20 to 30 seconds. If something feels good, and you feel that you're making progress, by all means, hold it for longer. I suggest you do at least two sets on each side; this extra set can really increase your range of motion.

Quadriceps Stretch

Stand, supporting yourself with one hand on a chair or other surface. Hold the outside of your foot, and gently pull your heel toward your buttock until you feel a stretch in the front of your thigh.

Hold for 20 to 30 seconds. Repeat twice on both sides.

CHALLENGE YOURSELF!

To add a balance component to this stretch, let go of the support and place the hand that's not holding the foot on your hip.

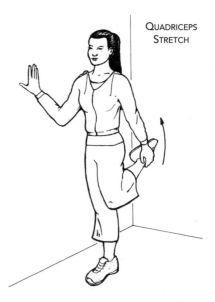

QUADRICEPS
STRETCH

Hamstring Stretch

Lie on your back with your knees bent and your feet on the floor. Slip your towel behind the ball of one foot, and gently extend your leg until it is straightened, not locked, and the towel is taut. Move your foot above your head until you feel the stretch in the back of your thigh.

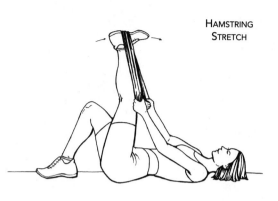

HAMSTRING STRETCH

Hold for 20 to 30 seconds. Repeat twice on both sides.

CHALLENGE YOURSELF!

If you'd like a slightly deeper stretch, extend the bottom leg so that it's flat on the ground. Keep both hips evenly weighted on the ground.

Hip Flexor Stretch

Kneel with one foot on the ground and one knee on a towel folded to create a pad. Keeping your body upright, lean your weight forward so that you can feel a stretch from your abs, through your hip flexor, to your thigh.

The knee of the front foot should never be farther forward than your toes.

Hold for 20 to 30 seconds. Repeat twice on both sides.

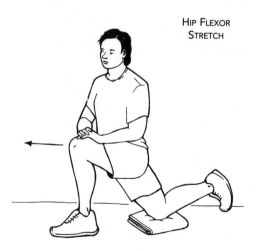

HIP FLEXOR STRETCH

Piriformis Stretch

This is a difficult muscle group to stretch properly, which makes this a great stretch.

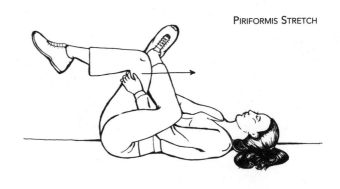

PIRIFORMIS STRETCH

Lie on your back with your knees bent and your feet on the floor. Cross your legs at the knees with the side you're stretching on top. While grasping the back of your bottom thigh with both hands, gently pull that bottom knee toward the shoulder on the same side as the bottom leg until a stretch is felt in the buttock and hip area.

Hold for 20 to 30 seconds. Repeat twice on both sides.

Iliotibial Band Stretch

Cross your left foot over your right foot with your right hand on the wall and your left hand on your hip. Lean your right hip to the wall while bending your left knee, keeping the right knee straight until you can feel a stretch in your right hip. For a variation on this stretch, cross your left foot behind the right.

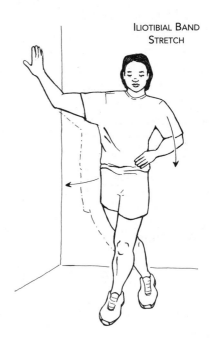

ILIOTIBIAL BAND STRETCH

Hold for 20 to 30 seconds. Repeat twice on both sides.

Note: The iliotibial band is difficult to stretch. Even if you feel this stretch only at the top of the hipbone, or in your abdominals, you will get a benefit from doing it.

Calf Stretch

Place both hands on the wall at shoulder height, and move one leg behind the other. The front leg should be bent, while the back leg stays straight with the heel on the ground and the toes turned outward a little. Lean forward into the wall until you feel the stretch in your calf.

Hold for 20 to 30 seconds. Repeat twice on both sides.

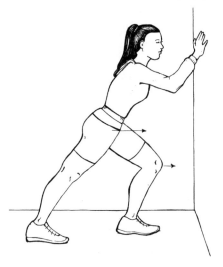

CALF STRETCH

Strengthening Exercises

You'll find the corresponding exercises for the following workouts in the section that follows.

GENERAL KNEE HEALTH WORKOUT

Quad Set
Straight Leg Raise with
  Rotation
Terminal Knee Extension
Hip Abduction
Inner Thigh Lift
Wall Slide
One Foot Balance
Leg Press with Ball Squeeze
Leg Curl
Partial Quadriceps Extension
Inner Thigh Squeeze

ACL HEALTH WORKOUT

Straight Leg Raise with
  Rotation
Hip Abduction
Hip Extension
Step Up
Step Down
Wall Slide
One Foot Balance
Tip Toes
Leg Press with Ball Squeeze
Leg Curl

PATELLOFEMORAL HEALTH WORKOUT

Quad Set
Straight Leg Raise with
  Rotation
Terminal Knee Extension
Inner Thigh Lift
One Foot Balance
Tip Toes
Leg Press with Ball Squeeze
Leg Curl
Inner Thigh Squeeze

"ON THE RUN" STRETCHING AND STRENGTHENING WORKOUT

Quadriceps Stretch
Hamstring Stretch
Hip Flexor Stretch
Straight Leg Raise
  with Rotation
Terminal Knee Extension
Wall Slide

CORE STRENGTH WORKOUT

Bridge with Ball
Modified Crunch
Bent Knee Lift
Leg Press with Ball Squeeze

The Equipment You'll Need

You don't need expensive workout aids to get a great knee workout.
Here's what you'll need:

- Towel

- Rubber ball or yoga block

- Six-inch step—anything stable, like a small box or a stool, or
  even a big dictionary will do.

LET'S GET TO WORK!

Quad Set

Focus: Inner and outer quadriceps strength and timing

Sit up, with a flat back and your legs extended in front of you. Place a rolled towel underneath the knee you're working on. Push the back of your knee into the towel, *keeping the heel down and in contact with the floor.* Hold for 10 seconds, release, and repeat.

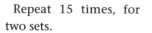
QUAD SET

Repeat 15 times, for two sets.

CHALLENGE YOURSELF!

Add 15 to 20 seconds for another two sets.

Straight Leg Raise with Rotation

Focus: Hip flexors, inner quad (VMO) strength, and timing

Recline, so that you're leaning on your elbows. The leg you're working is extended in front of you, the other is bent so that your foot is on the floor. Flex the working foot up so the foot is flat and *turn it* slightly (your right foot will be pointing to one o'clock when you're working that leg; your left foot will point to eleven). Tighten the muscle at the top of the thigh, and lift your leg almost parallel to the opposite knee. Hold for 3 seconds, return the leg to the ground with control, and repeat.

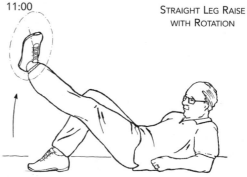
11:00
STRAIGHT LEG RAISE WITH ROTATION

Repeat 15 times, for two sets.

CHALLENGE YOURSELF!

Sit up with a flat back and lean back on your hands. Raise your leg as described above.

Repeat 15 times, for two sets.

Terminal Knee Extension

Recline, so that you're leaning on your elbows, with your legs extended in front of you. Place two rolled towels (or a rubber ball) under the knee you're working. Push the back of your knee into the towels or ball so that your heel comes up off the floor. Hold for 2 seconds, release, and repeat. Repeat 15 times, for two sets.

Challenge Yourself!

Add an ankle weight to the working leg.

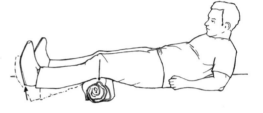

TERMINAL KNEE EXTENSION

Bridge with Ball

Focus: Build core strength, lower back, buttocks

Lie on your back with your knees bent so that your feet are flat on the floor. Place a block or ball between your thighs. Keeping your shoulders on the floor and underneath your body, raise your hips. Hold the position for 2 to 3 seconds, lower your pelvis to the ground with control, and repeat. Repeat 15 times, for two sets.

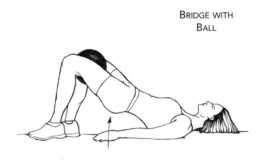

BRIDGE WITH BALL

Note: if you have a history of lower back pain, consult your doctor before doing this exercise.

Modified Crunch

Focus: Build core strength, abdominal muscles

Lie on your back with your legs bent, so your heels are in contact with the ground. Hold a ball above your face, so that your arms are directly in line with the shoulders. Lift your shoulder blades off the ground, *keeping your arms straight and the ball directly above your eyes.* Resist the temptation to bring the ball forward. Don't crane your neck, which will bring it out of alignment with the rest of your body. Hold for 3 seconds, lower your upper body to the ground with control, and repeat.

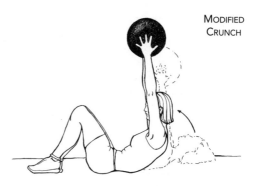

MODIFIED CRUNCH

Start with 15, and build up to two to three sets over a couple of weeks.

CHALLENGE YOURSELF!

Raise your entire upper body off the floor, keeping the ball above your eyes. Your feet should never leave the ground.

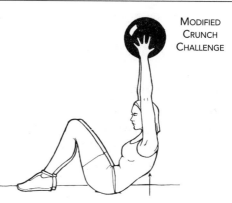

MODIFIED CRUNCH CHALLENGE

Start with 15, and build up to two to three sets over a couple of weeks.

Hip Abduction

Focus: Outside hip

HIP ABDUCTION

Lie on your side, with your legs extended. You can prop your head up with your arm. Tighten the thigh of the top leg and then lift that leg 8 to 10 inches, keeping the

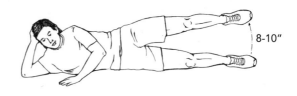

8-10"

foot parallel to the floor. (Keep the bottom hipbone touching the ground, and don't allow your body to tip over to the front or the back.) Hold the leg up for 2 to 3 seconds, return the foot to the top of the bottom foot with control, and repeat. Repeat 15 times, for two sets.

Hip Extension

Focus: Hamstring, buttocks, lower back strength

Lie on your stomach, with your legs extended. Lift the working leg 4 to 6 inches off the ground. (Keep both of your hipbones securely rooted to the floor—don't roll onto the nonworking side.) Hold for 2 to 3 seconds, return the leg to the ground with control, and repeat. Repeat 15 times, for two sets.

Note: If you're feeling low back pain when you do this exercise, you may be raising your leg too high.

HIP EXTENSION

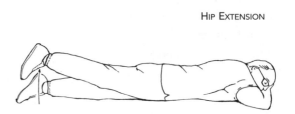

Bent Knee Lift

Focus: Core strength, buttocks, lower back

Lie on your stomach with your nonworking leg extended, and your working leg bent at a 90-degree angle. Cushion your head with your arms, and raise the bent leg. Hold for 2 to 3 seconds, return the knee to the ground with control, and repeat.

Repeat 15 times, for two sets.

BENT KNEE LIFT

Note: If you're feeling lower back pain when you do this exercise, you may be raising your leg too high.

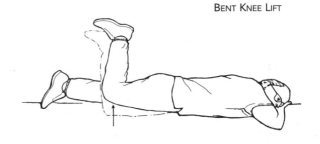

Inner Thigh Lift

Focus: Inner thigh strength

Lie on your side. The top leg is the nonworking leg, and should be crossed in front of or behind the working leg, so that the foot of the nonworking leg is on the ground. Contract the inner thigh, and raise the working leg about six inches off the ground. Hold for 3 seconds, return the leg to the ground with control, and repeat.

Make sure you're lying on a comfortable, lightly padded surface (a towel or rug on the floor will do), or this exercise may be uncomfortable for the hip.

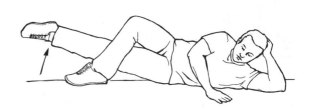

INNER THIGH LIFT

Repeat 15 times, for two to three sets.

Note: If you have an MCL injury, you should not do this exercise.

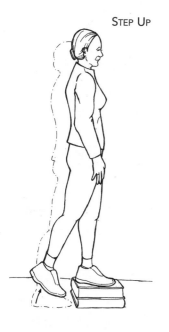

STEP UP

Step Up

Focus: VMO, inner and outer quad strength, timing, proprioception, and kinesthetic awareness

Stand facing your step, and step up with the working leg, moving the weight from your heel to your toe. Keep your weight on the working leg, push off from it, not the back leg, and slowly bring the other foot up without placing it on the step, so you're balancing on the working leg. Hold the balance for 3 seconds, return the nonworking leg to the ground, step off the step slowly with the working leg, and repeat.

Repeat 15 times, for two sets.

CHALLENGE YOURSELF!

Increase the amount of time you can hold the balance, up to 30 seconds. For an extra boost, hold a set of dumbbells by your side as you work. Beginners can add between 3 and 8 pounds, intermediates can add 5 to 15 pounds, and advanced people can add between 15 and 30.

Step Down

Focus: Eccentric/deceleration muscle strength, quadriceps strength, proprioception, kinesthetic awareness

Stand with both feet on your step. Step down to the ground with the working leg, slowly, to the count of six. Then return the working foot back to the step to a count of three, and repeat.

Repeat 12 to 15 times. Work your way up to two or three sets over a period of weeks.

CHALLENGE YOURSELF!

Increase the amount of time it takes you to lower your foot, up to 10 seconds.

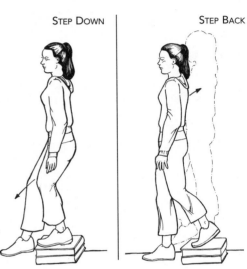

STEP DOWN   STEP BACK

A Word About Squats

Squats are some of the best all-around strength and conditioning exercises for the lower body. They're also some of the most misunderstood, by health professionals and patients alike.

It's true about all exercises, but especially squats: proper mechanics lead to results, poor mechanics lead to injury. I'm here to tell you that a properly executed squat is one of the safest exercises out there, and if you can remember to do the following, you'll be in good shape:

Keep your body in alignment. There should be a straight line from the top of your head through your shoulders, hips, knees, and heels.

You should never feel pain. If something hurts, you're doing it wrong. Check your alignment and decrease your range of motion (don't squat down as far). You should feel as if your muscles are working, however.

Bend from the hips—not from the knees. This isn't a complicated move, but it does have to be a conscious process. As you go down in your squat, think about flexing your hips, and allow your knees to bend automatically as a result of the hip flexion, instead of initiating the squat with the knees themselves. You'll feel the difference immediately.

If you have patellofemoral problems, begin if you are pain-free to 45 degrees and only progress up to 70 degrees if you stay pain-free. Decrease the range of motion slightly, so that you're better able to protect the joint. You'll still get all the quad strengthening benefit without the risk of aggravating your injury.

Don't permit your kneecaps to move out past your toes. If you're bending too deeply and putting too much weight into the front of your

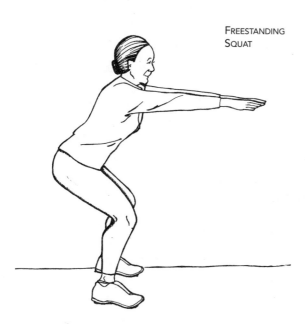

FREESTANDING
SQUAT

body, you're putting too much pressure on the front of the knees, and you're going to cause injury, not prevent or rehab it. Keeping your weight in your heels should help.

There's a quick test you can use to tell whether or not you're doing your squat correctly: you should always be able to look down and see your toes peeking out below your knees. If your knees are blocking the view, your feet are too far back.

If you follow these simple rules, you'll be able to avail yourself of the benefits of these wonderful, all-over leg-conditioning exercises with none of the negative consequences of doing them incorrectly.

Wall Slide

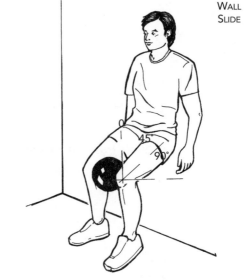

WALL SLIDE

Focus: Inner and outer quad strength, hamstring, core strength. abdominals, and buttocks

Stand with your back against a wall. With your feet parallel to each other, and gripping a block or a ball between your knees, slide down the wall until your knees bend at about a 45-degree angle. Don't let your knees go past your toes. Hold for 15 seconds.

Repeat 10 times, for two sets.

CHALLENGE YOURSELF!

Move your feet out so that you can slide down the wall until your thighs are parallel to the floor. Don't let your knees go past your toes. To increase the challenge even further, increase the length of time you hold the stretch, up to 60 seconds. Repeat 5 times, for two to three sets.

And before you complain: professional skiers routinely hold this version of the exercise for *ten whole minutes*, every time they train!

BALANCE

One Foot Balance

Focus: Balance, foot and ankle strength

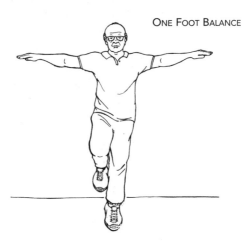

ONE FOOT BALANCE

If you have an injury, practice first on the noninjured leg. With your arms out to the side, stand on one leg. Looking straight ahead at a fixed spot, hold for up to 30 seconds. Release. Repeat on the other side.

Repeat 8 to 10 times.

CHALLENGE YOURSELF!

To really test your balance, put your hands on your hips. Hold the balance for a minute on each side. For a super challenge, close your eyes.

Tip Toes

Focus: Calf muscles, balance

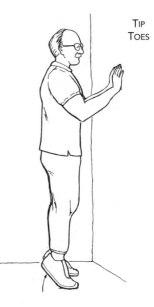

TIP TOES

Stand with your feet hip-width apart, toes turned slightly out. Raise yourself up on the balls of your feet and hold the position for 3 seconds. Lower your heels to the ground and repeat. If you're having difficulty with balance, keep your gaze on a fixed point straight ahead of you. Repeat 15 times, for two sets.

CHALLENGE YOURSELF!

Start in the same position, but with your knees slightly bent (as with all squats, they shouldn't go past your toes). Straighten

your knees and raise yourself up on the
balls of your feet, hold the position for 3
seconds, and then softly drop back into
position with your knees bent. Repeat. For
an extra boost, hold a set of dumbbells by
your side as you work. Beginners can add
between 3 and 8 pounds, intermediates
can add 5 to 15 pounds, and advanced
people can add between 15 and 30. When
you've mastered this, do it with closed eyes!

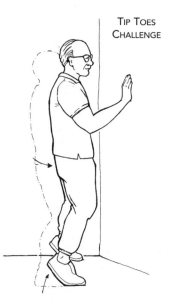

TIP TOES
CHALLENGE

EXERCISES WITH EQUIPMENT

The following exercises require equipment that is standard in most
gyms. You can begin these exercises after you've been doing the exercises
that don't require equipment for two to three weeks, three times a week.

If you don't have access to a gym, or if your gym doesn't have the
machines featured in these exercises, simply do another set of an exercise for the focus muscle group from the section above. If you do have
access to these machines, your workout only has three components:
stretching, balance, and exercises with equipment.

*Since everyone reading this will have a different strength level, I'm going
to use the words "medium," "medium hard," and difficult" to describe
the weight level you should use. An exercise is medium if you can get
through a set of 15, feeling the burn without being fatigued. It's "medium
hard" if you can get through the last rep of the set, but just barely. It's
"difficult" if you begin to fail on the last rep or two.*

Leg Press with Ball Squeeze

Focus: Quadriceps, buttocks, hamstring, eccentric quad contractions

Lie on a leg press machine, with your feet parallel to each other and high up on the platform, squeezing a ball between your thighs. Push the platform until your legs are straight but not locked. Your knees should never be at more than a 90-degree angle. Release slowly and repeat.

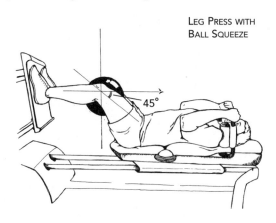

LEG PRESS WITH
BALL SQUEEZE

Do one set of 15, medium weight; one set of 15 medium-heavy weight.

> **Note**: If you have patellofemoral pain, begin pain-free to 45 degrees and progress up to 70 degrees (only as long as you stay pain-free).

CHALLENGE YOURSELF!

Concentric Set: Remove the ball, and do the exercise using a single leg at half the "medium" weight of your first set. Do one to two sets of 15.

Eccentric Set: Using medium weight, push the platform up with both legs to the count of three, and then lower the platform with just one leg, to the count of six. Do one to two sets of 15.

Leg Curl

Focus: Hamstring, eccentric contractions

Lie on your stomach on the leg curl machine. Bring your heels up so that your knees are bent to 90 degrees. Release slowly.

> **Note**: If you have a meniscal injury, stop at

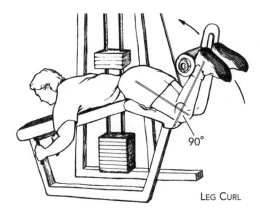

LEG CURL

70 to 80 degrees, or whatever angle allows you to do the exercise without pain.

Do one set of 15, medium weight; one set of 12 to 15, medium-heavy weight.

Partial Quadriceps Extension

Focus: Quadriceps, especially the VMO

Set the machine so that your lower legs are at a 45-degree angle to your thighs when you're in the starting position. Some machines allow you to change the starting position; otherwise you may have to raise the bar to 45 degrees yourself and make sure that it never drops below there. Sit in the chair, hooking your ankles behind the pads, and lift your legs to zero degrees. Keep your toes flexed. Release slowly and repeat.

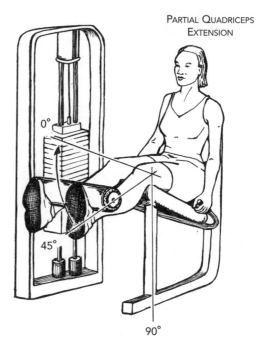

PARTIAL QUADRICEPS
EXTENSION

Do one set of 15, medium weight; one set of 12 to 15 medium-heavy weight.

CHALLENGE YOURSELF!

Do two sets, one medium and one medium hard, *using only one leg.*

Inner Thigh Squeeze

Focus: Inner thighs

Sit in the chair and set the machine so that your inner thighs feel stretched but not strained. Squeeze your inner thighs, moving your legs together. Hold for three seconds. Return weights to starting position as slowly as possible.

Note: If you have an MCL injury, you should not do this exercise.

Do one set of 15, medium weight; one set of 12 to 15 medium-heavy weight.

INNER THIGH SQUEEZE

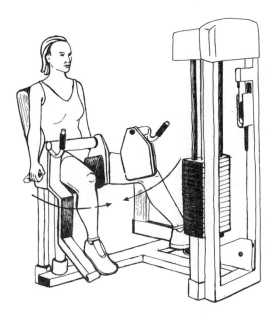

COMPLEMENTARY MEDICINE

A mericans spend billions of dollars a year on so-called alternative therapies: dietary supplements, homeopathy, traditional Chinese medicine. At least once a day, one of the patients in my practice asks me to weigh in on one of these alternatives.

Rather than alternatives, I prefer to think of these therapies as *complementary* to the Western-style medicine I'm doling out. The two systems aren't mutually exclusive; in fact, when you combine a dietary supplement with an NSAID and a program of quad-strengthening exercises, you're getting the best of both worlds.

For help with this chapter, I turned to a friend and fellow physician who has been practicing the ancient Chinese medical tradition of acupuncture for thirty-odd years. I've been referring patients interested in exploring acupuncture to him for years, but this book gave us a chance to talk about our medical philosophies. I was pleased and surprised to realize just how much overlap there was. Many of the topics we covered in that first conversation about complementary medicine were some of the themes that motivated me to write this book in the first place.

For instance, the importance of balance. We know that it's essential to achieve a physical balance—many of the injuries we discuss in this book are directly linked to strength, flexibility, or timing imbalances between different parts of the body, or different parts of the leg itself. There needs to be a balance between your front and your back, your inside and your outside. Your physical sense of balance is one of the things you lose when you get injured; and you'll find that many of the exercises in our workouts are designed to help you hone or regain your balance. We've also talked about the importance of finding a balance between exercise and rest: why it's so important that your training schedule include a day or two of rest per week, and how important it is to negotiate a compromise between keeping the joint mobile and not overtaxing an already weakened joint.

This concept of balance is also central to many of the alternative therapies my patients use to cope with their pain. For instance, acupuncture is based on the theory that illness and injury are caused by a result of a blockage in the energy force that moves through the body. When that blockage is removed, the body can come back into balance and heal itself, which is its natural inclination anyway.

We also spoke about the importance of building the person, instead of just attacking the complaint. The Western model of medicine is more disease-oriented, while the Chinese model focuses on building up the immune system and working preventively from within. This should sound familiar. I've said over and over again that having a strong, flexible, well-balanced leg capable of withstanding the pressures you put on it is one of the best defenses against knee pain and injury. It's a much more prevention-oriented approach.

I've also talked about the importance of treating the *whole* patient, not just "a knee" or an MRI. In 1911, Sir William Osler said, "It is much more important to know what sort of *patient* has a disease than what sort of disease a person has." The state of someone's marriage, their financial situation, the stresses and imbalances in their lives as a whole—these things can have as much bearing on their knee health as their tendency to pronate. This is a very real part of going to see a good alternative therapist: it's an integrative way of looking at a patient, one that encompasses the physical, the emotional, and the spiritual, and addresses these aspects equally.

We also discussed the importance, in both of our traditions, of encouraging patients to be active participants in their own recovery. People go to an alternative practitioner because they are taking responsibility for their pain or injury and actively looking for a solution to that problem. This is the same thing that makes physical therapy successful. A sports physician or physical therapist can only take you part of the way there: it's the extra mile—the effort you put in even though it hurts, the home therapy session you do before work even though you'd rather have another half hour in bed—that makes the difference between a brilliantly successful recovery and an injury that lingers.

In short, as Sir William Osler knew, much of what makes a good alternative therapist is plain old good doctoring.

Now here's my disclaimer: there's just not a whole lot of science behind many of the treatments and therapies described in this chapter. Big studies are expensive, and in many cases the supplement companies and complementary practitioners have not been able to devote the money to these projects. There's a difference in philosophy as well. Let's say you go to see an acupuncturist for knee pain. Your knee pain is somewhat alleviated, and you find yourself getting fewer urinary tract infections, and lower blood pressure to boot. At the end of a year, you require knee surgery. Was the acupuncture a failure? You certainly wouldn't say so, but a randomized, placebo-controlled double blind study might.

I can only give you a sampling of what's out there and let you know when I've seen overwhelmingly good results in my patients. If I haven't seen good results, or any results at all, or if in my opinion the science isn't there yet, I'll say that too. If there's one thing I do know, it's that many of these treatments seem to work idiosyncratically: a real pain breakthrough for one person will bounce off another with no effect at all. It will take work (and perhaps some money) to discover what works best for you.

Ultimately, the decision to pursue these therapies is one for you to make with your doctor. Please don't undertake any of the following without getting his or her opinion.

Herbal Supplements

Herbs and various plant extracts have been used for thousands of years to treat a wide variety of conditions and diseases. That means that there's a great deal of anecdotal evidence to support the claims made on their behalf. Dietary supplements are anything taken orally to supplement the diet. (Some of these treatments are not appropriate for oral consumption.)

A word of warning: Vitamins, minerals, and herbs aren't harmless simply because they're "natural" products—as a spokesperson for the FDA famously said, poisonous mushrooms are "natural," too. Just because you can buy these products over-the-counter doesn't mean that you should take them without medical supervision. Before you start taking any supplement, please discuss the specific supplement *and dosage* with your doctor.

It's important to remember that we don't have either the safety or efficacy data on supplements that we do on the FDA-approved drugs. Supplements can be toxic in the incorrect dosage, they can react badly with other medications you're taking, and they can have harmful effects on other aspects of your health.

ARNICA

Arnica comes from the head of a yellow flower and has been used as a homeopathic preparation for hundreds of years. It is believed to stimulate white blood cell activity, reducing inflammation; in fact, many commercially available liniments include it. It is available as a cream and as a homeopathic remedy for oral consumption.

BOSWELLA OR BOSWELLIA

Derived from tree resin, this herbal remedy has been used for centuries as a home remedy in India. It is believed to have an anti-inflammatory effect and is used primarily by people with osteoarthritis and rheumatoid arthritis. Those who have had good results with this herb believe that it relieves swelling and pain, lessens morning stiffness, and promotes joint function.

BUYER BEWARE!

Supplements aren't regulated by the Federal Drug Administration (FDA). Because of that, there's often a lack of consistency in the way they're manufactured, which in turn has an effect on their potency and efficacy, so you may want to stick with a major brand, or ask your doctor to recommend a specific company. Look for "standardized extract"— it's not a guarantee (it simply means that the preparation is standard within the company), but it's better than nothing.

One more thing to think about before you begin pursuing supplementation therapy: cost. Some of these supplements are relatively expensive, and you have to take a lot of them (especially if you're managing chronic pain), so that may be a consideration in your decision to pursue this path.

Scientists believe that boswella's effectiveness has to do with its ability to suppress leukotrienes, the cells that promote inflammation, by blocking their synthesis. It may also contain agents that increase the blood flow to the joint.

In rare cases, boswella may cause gastrointestinal distress or a skin rash. If you begin experiencing side effects, stop taking the herb immediately.

It is available both in pill form and as a topical cream. Look for products standardized to 60 percent boswellic acids, and if you're taking it orally, discuss dosages with your doctor.

CHINESE THUNDER GOD VINE (LEI GONG TENG OR TRIPTERYGIUM WILFORDII)

What a name! Although the leaves and flowers of this plant are extremely toxic, the roots reduced pain and swelling in people with rheumatoid arthritis in a small study funded by the National Institute of Arthritis and Musculoskeletal and Skin Diseases and published in the journal *Arthritis & Rheumatism.*

It's believed to be an anti-inflammatory and may also retard an overactive immune system—the cause of rheumatoid arthritis. This root appears to be well tolerated, although gastrointestinal distress was experienced by one person who participated in the study, and there have also been reports of reversible male infertility.

I'm hesitant to recommend anything that has the potential to be this toxic. If you are interested in pursuing this herb anyway, please be careful about preparing this root as a tea by yourself: its other folk name is "Walk Seven Steps and Die" because the flowers are so poisonous.

ENZYMES

An Austrian study, which was published in the journal *Clinical Drug Investigation*, found that a combination of bromelain, trypsin, and rutin was as effective as the NSAID diclofenac in patients with osteoarthritis of the knee.

Early studies indicate that naturally derived enzymes can have both an analgesic and an anti-inflammatory effect.

These should not be taken by people who are also using blood-thinning medication such as coumadin.

Glucosamine and Chondroiten Sulfate

These two supplements are naturally occurring cartilage building blocks and may contribute to the repair and maintenance of healthy cartilage; glucosamine may also block cartilage-destroying enzymes. The groundswell about these supplements started in 1997, with the publication of the bestseller, *The Arthritis Cure,* by Dr. Jason Theodosakis.

These supplements may not be a cure, but there is certainly a wealth of anecdotal evidence, including in my own practice, that they work. The anecdotal evidence has been compelling enough to catch the attention of the medical establishment. In March 2000, the prestigious *Journal of the American Medical Association (JAMA)* published an article that summed up a number of the studies that had been done on glucosamine and chondroiten and their effect on osteoarthritis sufferers. The *JAMA* report concluded that, even though many of the studies were small and badly designed, both glucosamine and chondroiten sulfate did have a beneficial effect on pain and joint mobility.

More answers are coming. The National Institute of Health is currently sponsoring a large clinical trial to look at the effects of these supplements on osteoarthritis of the knee. The study will look at more than 1,000 patients on a six- and eighteen-month treatment regimen; preliminary results are expected in March 2005, so stay tuned.

People who have had good experiences with these supplements claim that they are at least as effective as ibuprofen at relieving pain, and some studies have shown that they may even prevent further degeneration in the joint.

These supplements are generally well-tolerated, although there are some concerns about the interactions of chondroiten sulfate with blood-thinning medications like coumadin, but with pure products, this is less likely. Care should be taken in the diabetic patient, and if you're allergic to shellfish, you should seriously consider not taking these supplements.

My patients have received relief from these supplements, and they're something I do recommend. If you suffer from osteoarthritis, or if you're at elevated risk because of a previous injury, like an meniscal tear, or a chronic knee condition like patellofemoral disorder, I strongly suggest that you discuss the possibility of pursuing these supplements with your doctor.

GINGER (ZINGIBER OFFICINALE)

Ginger is the root of a flower belonging to the lily family, and it's one of the most commonly used ingredients in Chinese and Indian food.

Herbally, it's mainly used as a tonic to soothe nausea, but it has also been used in the Indian Ayurvedic system as an anti-inflammatory, and is a new favorite among people with rheumatoid and osteo-arthritis who are looking to control their swelling and chronic pain. Proponents claim that it's as effective as an over-the-counter NSAID without the gastrointestinal side effects, although it may cause gastrointestinal distress if you take a very high dose.

It's available in the form of capsules, tea, and, of course, the raw herb—though the dosage you get in the less concentrated forms may not be high enough. Look for "standardized extract," and talk to your doctor about how much you'll need to take to see a difference in your swelling and discomfort.

GREEN TEA

It has been shown that green tea, which is widely drunk in many Asian countries, has a high level of antioxidants. An animal study funded by the Arthritis Foundation has shown that mice who were given green tea extracts developed less rheumatoid arthritis and milder cases of the disease than those not given green tea.

There don't seem to be any side effects at all to green tea, even when taken in relatively large doses, but it does contain caffeine. If you're caffeine-sensitive, you can try a decaffeinated brand.

MSM

Methylsulfonylmethane, known as MSM, is a supplemental form of dietary sulphur, the sulphur ordinarily found in many different types of food, but destroyed when those foods are processed.

The jury is still out on this one for me: although there are people lined up to tout this supplement (including the late actor James Coburn, who claimed it allowed him to return to acting despite disabling rheumatoid arthritis), there's almost no hard science to support it. There's certainly no science to support the claim that it fixes or protects cartilage.

This supplement appears to be well tolerated, although caution should be taken if you're contemplating surgery, have an existing bleeding disorder, or are taking a blood-thinning medication like coumadin. Like all supplements, you should discuss use with your doctor, especially if you're using other medications.

OMEGA-3 FATTY ACIDS

Omega-3s, the oils found in coldwater fatty fish like salmon, mackerel, and tuna, are the supplement stars of the cardiology world for their ability to lower triglycerides and confer other heart-healthy benefits.

But before they were used to promote heart health, omega-3s were used to promote joint health. There are records of arthritic patients being dosed with codliver oil as early as the late 1700s. Researchers believe that these oils can reduce inflammation and may prevent the disintegration of cartilage. Their theory is somewhat borne out by the fact that people who live in cultures with a fish-heavy diet have fewer rheumatic problems. The use of omega-3s to reduce pain and inflammation has been endorsed by the Arthritis Foundation.

So should you eat more fish? Yes—because it's good for you, and lower in both fat and calories than red meat, which can help with weight control (always a good idea for your knees). But you probably can't get enough omega-3s to be beneficial for your joints through your diet alone, so you may want to discuss a supplement with your doctor.

Because these omega-3s act as blood thinners, they should not be used by anyone contemplating surgery, with an existing bleeding disorder, or anyone taking a blood-thinning medication like coumadin. They also need to be taken in relatively large doses to be effective, which causes some people gastrointestinal distress.

NETTLE LEAF

Also called stinging nettle, this plant has stinging thorns. Gardeners with arthritis often go right to the source and just sting themselves with the nettle plant itself. Widely used in Europe, this Native American remedy for arthritis seems to have anti-inflammatory effects. There have even been small studies demonstrating that nettle leaf allowed arthritis sufferers to cut back on their NSAID dose, and one that showed that taking nettle in combination with the anti-inflammatory drug diclofenac enhanced the effects of that drug.

Both nettle root and nettle leaf are available, but it seems to be nettle *leaf* that has the positive effects for arthritis sufferers. It's available orally and as a topical cream.

SHARK CARTILAGE

This supplement, made from the skeletal material of sharks, came to prominence as a "cure" for cancer—a claim that resulted in a lawsuit by the FDA against the company promoting it. It has since found favor among arthritis sufferers for reducing joint inflammation and the pain associated with it.

Sharks do get cancer, and they don't have knees. I don't have a lot of experience with this through my patients, and I'm unconvinced by the scientific data on it thus far. It does contain high levels of chondroiten, which I do believe has pain-lessening effects for some people, but I'm not sure that there are additional benefits to be gained from this supplement.

WHITE WILLOW BARK (SALIX ALBA)

White willow bark has been used to relieve pain and fever for hundreds of years. The leaves, which can be chewed, are the source of one of our most commonly used and effective medications, salicylic acid, the leading ingredient in aspirin.

Many people who have difficulty taking aspirin because of sensitive stomachs or ulcers often have no such difficulty with white willow bark. If you have these difficulties, it's a good idea to check with your doctor before taking white willow bark, and anyone with a known allergy to aspirin should avoid it altogether.

Massage

I'm using massage as an umbrella term here. There are literally hundreds of varieties of soft tissue manipulation by a practitioner, varying from a sports-oriented massage by a physical therapist to a laying-on of hands by a Reiki master.

Many of my patients get massages as often as they can find the time and money to do so. Massage can help to improve circulation and relax muscles, lower blood pressure, and increase range of motion. It's not clear whether or not there are long-term benefits, but the short-term ones are clear: massage feels good, and that can be a real boon to someone with knee pain, or coping with soreness after athletics, or dealing with the chronic pain of arthritis.

And don't rule out self-massage! It is our first instinct—when something hurts, rub it. You can massage yourself with your bare hands, an inexpensive vibrating wand available at a drugstore—even a tennis ball rolled on the painful area can help. And while your partner may not be officially licensed to practice massage, someone else's touch can be a welcome respite from the pain.

GIVING A MASSAGE TO SOMEONE SUFFERING FROM KNEE PAIN

Giving a massage doesn't have to be a big deal, with a padded table and aromatherapy and warmed towels. A five-minute rub while you're both watching television can be beneficial to someone struggling with knee pain from an injury or arthritis, especially after a period of difficult activity.

Make sure the person is in a comfortable position. It'll make it easier for them to relax.

Use a lubricant so your skin doesn't drag against theirs. Massage oil stays slippery longer without getting sticky, but any moisturizer will do. You may want to mix in a little liniment as well.

Massage not only the muscles immediately in the area of pain, but the muscles that feed into it. Massaging the hip, the calves, the ankles and feet, and the lower back can alleviate a great deal of knee pain.

Use the pads of your fingers, not the tips, and be sensitive to the response you're getting. A touch that is too light may cause a tickle response, and going too deep may cause pain. Bear in mind that some places may be sorer than others, and less tolerant to deep touch. It's useful to remember that you're massaging muscle—not skin, and not bone.

Everyone likes to be touched differently—sometimes the same person has different requests and requirements on different days! You'll get a feeling for what feels good as you continue to experiment.

FINDING A MASSAGE PRACTITIONER

Your physical therapist or doctor may be able to recommend a massage therapist, and your insurance may even cover part of it if your doctor prescribes it for you. Licensed massage therapists will refer to themselves as such, and will have passed a state examination (most states have one).

Before you see someone for a massage, it's a good idea to ask what techniques are used, what that means, and whether or not the therapist has had experience with your particular problem before.

The American Massage Therapy Association (AMTA) "works to establish massage therapy as integral to the maintenance of good health and complementary to other therapeutic practices." It requires members to have at least 500 hours of training, and hosts a list of member practitioners on its website: *www.amtamassage.org* or you can call toll-free: 888-843-2682.

The National Certification Board for Therapeutic Massage and Bodywork is a private, nonprofit organization that offers credentials to massage therapists after they've proven to have a certain level of training and experience. It holds its members to a code of ethics and professional standards. You can find a nationally certified therapist on their website, *www.ncbtmb.com*, or you can call for information: 703-610-0281.

MASSAGE TECHNIQUES

Even under the umbrella term of conventional massage, there is a wide range of techniques and philosophies. You may have to experiment to discover which one works for you. Some people love a deep massage, while it's torture for others. Some people are soothed by more gentle treatments, and others don't feel they do anything. Much depends on the way you like to be touched, and the nature of your pain or injury.

HOW TO GET THE MOST OUT OF YOUR MASSAGE

— Arrive in plenty of time for your appointment. You'll want a moment to change and relax before the massage begins.

— Eating right before a massage isn't recommended.

— Talk to your practitioner. Tell him or her your medical diagnosis, where your pain is, what your preferences are. Although you may prefer to be quiet during the massage, you should feel free to speak up if something is uncomfortable or if something environmentally (the temperature, music volume) is bothering you.

— Don't forget to breathe!

Acupuncture

A major branch of traditional Chinese medicine, acupuncture, has been practiced in China for thousands of years. It involves the insertion of hair-thin needles into various points of the body to release the qi (pronounced chi), or life force, which causes pain and injury when blocked. Acupuncturists quote an ancient saying: "There is no illness except stagnation, no cure only the reestablishment of flow." The needles reestablish the flow, allowing the body to heal itself.

A 1998 study at Harvard estimated that Americans made over five million visits a year to acupuncturists—and that number has only grown since then. The World Health Organization recommends it for a variety of conditions, including rheumatoid arthritis, and the National Institute of Health claims that it "may be useful as an adjunct treatment or an acceptable alternative or be included in a comprehensive management program" for osteoarthritis and other conditions. Many of my patients use it to manage their pain, whether that pain is the result of trauma, surgery, or a chronic condition like arthritis.

There are few side effects associated with acupuncture. Some people report light-headedness after their first treatment. Most of the resistance to acupuncture is the fear factor: it's unsettling to imagine yourself as a human pincushion. But this is the last thing that those who have actually had the treatment complain about. Since the needles are so thin, there's usually only minimal discomfort when being treated by an experienced practitioner. The needles are sterile, and used one time only in order to eliminate the threat of infection or disease transmission.

Your doctor may, as I do, have an acupuncturist he feels comfortable referring patients to who are curious about this practice. If not, you can contact the American Association of Acupuncture and Oriental Medicine at 888-500-7999. You can find a referral to a physician with training in acupuncture from the American Academy of Medical Acupuncture, ***www.medicalacupuncture.com***, 800-521-2262.

Before you begin, ask your practitioner how many sessions you are likely to require, and the cost of each session. Your insurance company may cover part or all of the cost, but you should check before you begin treatment since many practitioner require preauthorization.

Magnets

An astonishing amount of anecdotal evidence supports the use of magnet therapy, much of it by star athletes, and a great number of my patients have benefited from this inexpensive treatment.

The science, as it is with most of the treatments in this chapter, is lagging behind, but there have been some compelling studies. One was done at the Baylor College of Medicine in 1997 by a cynic, Dr. Carlos Valbona, in post-polio patients and revealed a significant alleviation of pain in the magnet group. Another, published in *Alternative Therapies,* showed significant pain relief among people who suffer from osteoarthritis of the knee. But there have been other studies, including one done at the New York College of Podiatric Medicine, where both the magnetic and non-magnetic groups reported improvement. This may be attributed to the strength of the placebo effect. And a recent study, done at the University of Virginia and funded by a division of the NIH, published results in the *Journal of Alternative and Complementary Medicine* saying that although the results of the study were inconclusive, magnet therapy reduced fibromyalgia pain enough to be "clinically meaningful."

So it's up to you. Nobody really knows how it works; the science is lacking. People who have pacemakers or any kind of metal in their body should not use them.

When we talk about magnet therapy, we're not talking about the thing keeping the grocery list on the refrigerator. The strength of a magnet is measured in guass—a refrigerator magnet comes in at about 60 guass, while the magnets that are used for pain relief usually range between 300 and 4,000 guass. You can get them in braces, wraps, bracelets, even mattress pads. What appears to be more effective are larger magnets that you sit or lie in—these are presently being used throughout Europe.

Clearly more studies are needed to determine whether or not there are side effects, what conditions are likely to benefit most, and what strength of magnet is most efficacious.

Prolotherapy

Although it may seem counterintuitive, prolotherapy claims to stimulate the body's natural ability to heal itself by irritating it. In the same way that you encourage bone to grow stronger by putting stresses on it, or build muscle by breaking it down through exercise so it can grow back stronger, prolotherapists claim that by irritating soft tissue, you can goad it into regenerating itself. The "prolo" stands for proliferate.

A sugar water solution is injected into the damaged tissue, which causes an inflammation and increased blood supply to the area. A series of treatments are generally required (usually between four and ten) and it's common for people to experience soreness for a few days after the treatments. Because the point of the treatments is to encourage inflammation, NSAIDs aren't advised, but acetaminophen (Tylenol) can help relieve discomfort.

The science for prolotherapy is evolving. If you are interested or frustrated by no improvement in your symptoms with more conventional therapies, it may be worth discussing with your doctor.

THE PSYCHOLOGICAL EFFECTS OF KNEE INJURY

K nee pain and/or injury does not occur in a void—instead, it's the result of a cascade of events, which unfold with varying effects on mind, body, and spirit. Daily routines are altered, relationships temporarily change, coping mechanisms are activated—and all of this happens as you're trying to maintain both mental and physical function.

Much has been written about the psychological effects of injury on the professional or competitive athlete, and that's certainly a worthy topic. A knee injury can—and has, many times—ended a promising career. If your professional life depends on your body being in peak condition, then a knee injury, even a minor and treatable one, can be devastating psychologically. Your immediate performance is affected, and that injury also places your future potential in jeopardy, which can lead to increased anxiety and uncertainty for an athlete.

But it's not just pro players who suffer. As the title of this book suggests, when knee injury happens to you, it truly is a crisis. It affects your ability to move around, which is something we absolutely take for granted until it's taken away from us. If you have to take time off work to rest or heal after injury, it affects your income. If you have to pay for some or all of your treatment, it affects your pocketbook. If you have to postpone a trip to the zoo with your kids, or cancel a dancing lesson with your wife, it affects your family. If you have to cancel a vacation, it affects you socially. If you have to sit on the sidelines during your Wednesday night volleyball league game, it affects your conditioning. If you can't get up out of a chair after dinner without looking as if you're a million years old, it affects your self-image. If you're forced to assume a new dependence role on the people in your life, it can affect those relationships.

In other words, knee pain and injury can spur a whole series of transitions in your life, and these things conspire together to affect your mental health.

And often, the impact is felt long after the injury has healed. For instance, it's not unusual to feel that your body is untrustworthy. One of my patients confessed that she was having trouble dressing in the morning. Although her knee was perfectly stable, she felt too insecure about its capabilities to put all her weight on one leg, even for a moment. What a terrible, insecure way to start the day! The fear of re-injury runs deep, and it can make participation in sports, dancing, or activities of daily living difficult, giving rise to apprehension.

Obviously, there's no quick solution to these issues. But there are things you can do to help yourself. Countless studies have shown a strong connection between the mental and the physical: patients with a positive mental outlook recover faster and better than patients with negative outlooks. So it's in the interests of your knee as well as your emotional health that an important aspect of your rehab must address your emotional conditioning as well as your muscular strength.

Some things that have helped countless patients in the past:

Do something for your knee. A physical therapist once said to one of my discouraged patients: "The best thing you can do for your head right now is to do something for your knee." This is true for a number of reasons. First of all, you will feel better as you start to see progress in your healing, and the best way to do that is to actively participate in your rehabilitation. As your knee and leg get stronger, and as you begin to regain balance and coordination, you'll feel more confident about your body's abilities and less prone to re-injury. Of course, participation in exercise is associated with improved self-esteem, as well as reduced anxiety and depression. Take control of the process and do something about your recovery, and you'll feel better all around.

Manage your pain. Living in constant pain isn't necessary, and it can be emotionally draining, even resulting in serious depression if left unaddressed. Continue to discuss your medication options with your physician until you're both satisfied that your needs have been met. If you're uncomfortable taking medication to assist in pain control, then explore alternatives with your doctor and physical therapist.

Be patient. It's often true that the better you feel about your progress, the quicker you recover. Be realistic in your expectations. Begin with baby steps and small goal accomplishments: break up your recovery into small chunks. So, instead of worrying about next year's marathon, concentrate instead on meeting your targets at next week's stretching session. When you set realistic goals and meet them, you'll have a sense of accomplishment instead of having to cope with the immensity of the big picture.

Talk about it. Let your health care provider (doctor and physical therapist, and anyone else you may be seeing for your knee pain) know that you're having a hard time. Ask if they have any suggestions for you. You're definitely not alone, and they may be able to put you in touch with another patient or a group of people who have had similar issues. They also often have alternatives designed to improve your outcome and recovery. Use your everyday support system. Your parents, your spouse, your friends, your coaches, your teammates—anyone that you'd ordinarily talk to about a problem. An injury can be isolating, and going out for a cup of coffee with an old friend—even if the subject of your injury never comes up in any detail—can be helpful.

It can also be helpful to get some new perspectives on the potential and speed of your recovery. There are lots of websites hosting community message boards where you can post questions and meet people with similar injuries. It can be comforting to hear what worked for other people and to provide counsel and advice to others who are having a rough go of it. A word of warning: be careful about taking advice from strangers—there's a tremendous amount of misinformation out there, and anyone can have a medical degree if they're posting anonymously. Before you pursue any treatment modality, no matter how harmless it may seem, it's best to run it by your doctor. Of course, there are myriad mental health professionals who can help you as well.

Almost all active people become injured at some point in their lifetime, which means that almost all of us will be forced to deal with the physical, psychological, and social ramifications of injury at one point or another. Remember: your mental well-being has a direct affect on your physical recovery, so don't let it fall by the wayside.

PART V

GROUPS WITH SPECIAL CONCERNS

■ CHAPTER FIFTEEN ■

SPECIAL CONCERNS

Women

According to the American Academy of Orthopedic Surgeons, women are three to four times more likely to injure their knees than men playing the same sports. This is obviously of tremendous concern to active women, their coaches, and the physicians who treat them. Why are female athletes so at risk, and what can be done about it?

The most glaring example of the injury discrepancy between men and women is the anterior cruciate ligament, one of the bands that stabilize the knee. One study showed that women are up to eight times more likely to damage their ACLs than men. Female basketball players are twice as likely to damage their ACLs than their male counterparts, and female soccer players are four times more likely to sustain the injury.

This seems to be the result of an unfortunate combination of factors, the first of which is the anatomical difference between the sexes.

Anatomy

Women have a wider pelvis, so the thighbones come down at a sharper angle toward the shinbone. This results in a sharper quadriceps angle, known as the *Q angle*, which can cause the knee to bend inward. Wider hips place greater pressure on the inside of the knee.

The thighbone ends with two bumps (think of a dog's bone). The tunnel between those bumps is called the *intercondylar notch*. Women tend to have smaller, more narrow intercondylar notches, and the smaller the tunnel, the greater the chance of an ACL injury. If the tunnel is too narrow, then there's no room for the ACL to maneuver during a rapid cutting movement or sudden deceleration.

A smaller notch may also mean an ACL that didn't grow as large as it might have because of the bone surrounding it.

Hormones

Researchers are examining the link between female hormones and ACL injury. Female hormones allow for greater flexibility and looseness of muscles, tendons, and ligaments, and this looseness allows certain muscles and joints to withstand impact and damage, but it also transfers much of the force to the knee—especially the ACL.

The Estrogen Question

A study done at the University of Michigan found that women were almost three times as likely to injure their ACLs during ovulation than at other points during the cycle. Estrogen levels are higher during ovulation, and this may affect either the muscles, the ligaments, or the nervous system, making women more likely to sustain this injury in the middle of their cycle.

Because this increase was seen among women who were not using birth control pills, researchers suggested that oral contraceptives might offer a measure of protection against the injury, although there's certainly not enough evidence to support the use of the pill as a preventive measure against ACL injury.

Biomechanics

BENDING THE KNEES

Basketball and volleyball are sports that require a great deal of jumping—and landing from those jumps. These are the sports where most women hurt their ACLs.

Researchers now believe that the increased rate of injury has much to do with the way women play. They don't bend their knees and hips as much as men do when they land, which increases the force translated across the knee.

Soccer, basketball, and volleyball all require sudden changes in direction. Women tend to keep their knees and hips upright when they're pivoting, something else that puts a lot of pressure on the ACL. Women also tend to land on their toes, as opposed to rocking back onto their heels and allowing the back body to pick up some of the transferred forces.

When women are trained to land from a jump and flex their hips and knees, they suffer fewer ACL injuries.

BACK BODY STRENGTH

Women rely more on the strong muscles at the front of their body, like the quadriceps, than they do on the muscles at the back of the body, like the hamstrings. This is deadly in combination with their propensity to remain upright: if the knees aren't bent, overrelying on these strong muscles at the front of the body can result in damage to the ACL.

CONDITIONING

In the past, girls tended to get into sports later than boys, and they were often not as strong, fast, or coordinated as a result. The stresses that they put on their bodies in competitive sports are comparable, though, which may be why we see more injuries in girls and women.

Alison, 30

"I blew my ACL in January of 1990. I was seventeen years old, and it was the first game of my last varsity basketball season. I was starting center and co-captain, and in the best shape of my life.

The ACL happened in the first half, and I didn't even have the ball—I just twisted wrong, and I went down. I remember my coaches trying to reassure me as they helped me off the court, telling me that it was OK and that I'd be back in a couple of weeks, but I could tell from the looks on their faces that it was my last game of the season.

I was in surgery ten days later. I didn't have time to think about the long-term consequences—the six months of rehab in front of me, or my future in college sports. There was plenty of time to think later. I spent the next six weeks on crutches and the next six months in rehab. My whole life changed. Sports had been everything to me—the whole structure of my life. I was on three varsity teams, captain of two of them. I had morning practices, evening practices, weekend tournaments. I won the scholar-athlete award. My friends were all athletes. And their lives went on as usual while I was learning to walk again.

I'd missed the recruitment window for college volleyball, and although I showed up to the first tryout when I got to college, I wasn't on the radar, and it was pretty clear that they weren't interested. I'm pretty sure that I wasn't back to my preinjury level of play, either.

My whole life changed as a result of the ACL. I'm no longer "an athlete." I love the outdoors, and I love to Rollerblade and play tennis and swing dance and throw a Frisbee around, but it's not the way I identify myself. And my knee still hurts. I'm sure that some of that is because I'm not in the best shape I could be in, but it's still frustrating. I can't cross my legs for any period of time, for instance. If I do any kind of serious running, or play tennis for too long, it hurts. And my other knee is a problem waiting to happen, so I don't do anything that puts it in the line of fire, like skiing.

Ultimately, I'm not unhappy with the way things worked out—if I'd been a jock in college, I never would have discovered theater set design and carpentry, which are still very satisfying hobbies, and indirectly led me to a job I really enjoy. The thing I'm curious about is how a young female athlete in my shoes would be treated in 2003—and how she'll be treated in 2010. In 1990 it was pretty much a given that I would never have a college sports career, but I'd bet that's not true for a senior with a torn ACL now. I had a great rehab experience, but I certainly didn't do any sports-specific drills or training to get me back to my preinjury level. I'm sure that would be different now as well."

So what to do about the ACL epidemic in women's sports? Prevention, treatment, and rehabilitation for this injury is getting better and better. A female athlete with a torn ACL doesn't necessarily have to give it all up. The best course of preventive action would seem to be correcting muscular imbalances, improving agility, and other risk factors to the best of our abilities, and focusing on training female athletes with agility and landing drills that minimize their risk.

Pregnancy

During pregnancy, the body releases a hormone called relaxin, which encourages all the ligaments in the body to relax in order to prepare for labor. This loosening can be dangerous—the stabilizers supporting the knee are relaxing just at the point when a woman's center of gravity and balance systems are most unreliable.

You should discuss your exercise regime with your gynecologist or midwife over the course of your pregnancy; exercise may not be advised for everyone, and certain modifications may have to be made in your routine. No matter what, your body will require a little extra attention so you can protect yourself and your knees. You may find that you're more flexible than usual, so make sure not to overstretch. Your balance may be less sure than it is normally, so avoid or modify activities that put you at risk—you may want to do the step exercise class without a step, for instance. With a little additional care, you can exercise throughout your pregnancy without jeopardizing your knees.

The American College of Obstetrics and Gynecology has released guidelines for exercise in pregnancy. You can find it by searching "pregnancy exercise" in the patient education area of their website, *www.acog.org*.

The Female Athlete Triad

The female athlete triad is a combination of three major factors that puts some women at higher risk for certain injuries. These include stress fractures, as well as other injuries that may result from fatigue and low energy levels. The long-term effects of the triad may include bone loss and osteoporosis.

The three factors are an eating disorder, an infrequent or absent menstrual period, and bone loss.

Eating Disorders

This is a major issue for women, and women who participate in sports, especially sports where appearance is important, are especially at risk. We may think of the female athlete as the paragon of health, but the rate of eating disorders among young women who participate in sports tells us otherwise. Coaches and parents as well as participating athletes need to make sure that concentrating on performance and physical training does not result in an unhealthy obsession.

The two main eating disorders are bulimia and anorexia. Bulimia is a cycle of binging and purging. Anorexia is marked by adherence to a strict, extremely low-calorie diet. Both disorders may be accompanied by excessive exercise.

If left unaddressed, eating disorders can have devastating long-term effects on a woman's health and may even result in death. If you have an eating disorder, or if you suspect that someone you care about does, a number of resources can help, like the National Eating Disorders Association: *www.nationaleatingdisorders.org*, 800-931-2237.

AMMENORHEA

This is the absence of a menstrual period, and it generally signals a low estrogen level, which in turn is linked to lower bone mass. If a young woman has not gotten her first period by age sixteen, or if her period has stopped for more than three consecutive months due to excessive weight loss or exercise, she should see a doctor.

BONE LOSS

The lack of proper nutrition and the protective benefits of estrogen may result in bone loss, which can lead to bone weakness and a higher incidence of stress fracture. If left unaddressed, this condition may result in osteoporosis.

It is great to see the huge participation of women in sports in the twenty-first century. With this increasing participation, we're bound to see more injury—there are simply more athletes to get hurt. This increase is not only forcing doctors and researchers to become more aware of the differences between the sexes and how that manifests itself in injury profiles, but it's driving us to come up with better prevention and treatment options.

■ CHAPTER SIXTEEN ■

SPECIAL CONCERNS

Children

C hildren commonly develop knee problems, but it may be difficult for a parent to know when a child has a legitimate grievance about his or her knee. Children are very good at recruiting other structures to make up for pain or a loss of function in their knees, and they may not complain of pain until long after an adult would have.

A rule of thumb: kids don't usually fake a limp or an inability to play their favorite sport. If you suspect your child has knee pain, look out for limping, a tendency to favor one side, and a reduced interest in ordinarily pleasurable activities.

Some of the most common disorders causing knee pain in children follow.

Osgood-Schlatter's Disease

Osgood-Schlatter's disease, otherwise known as "growing pains," is caused by an irritation of the patellar tendon where it joins the shinbone. It is most often seen in active children.

The disease can be treated with relative rest, icing, compression, and bracing, although in rare cases immobilization is called for. This condition usually stops when the child stops growing, with no serious consequences for them as adults except a slightly enlarged bump on the front of the leg. For more information about Osgood-Schlatter's, please see pages 141-142.

Sinding-Larsen-Johansson Disease

Sinding-Larsen-Johansson disease is similar to Osgood-Schlatter's, but instead of manifesting where the patellar tendon joins the shinbone, the pain and irritation tend to be found where that tendon meets the patella. It causes swelling and pain, particularly after activity.

This condition is treated like Osgood-Schlatter's, with relative rest, icing, compression, and bracing, and like Osgood-Schlatter's, will usually resolve itself when the child stops growing.

Patellofemoral Syndrome

This is the most prevalent knee injury in children, especially active ones. It's an overuse injury, exacerbated by anatomical factors such as flatfeet and a large Q angle, and it manifests as pain under or around the kneecap, which gets worse with bent-leg activities such as squatting and stair climbing. Like adult patellofemoral syndrome, it's treated with relative rest, RICE, and taping or bracing, as well as a program to strengthen the knee.

It's important not to ignore signs of patellofemoral problems in your child. The child may need orthotics, or to stretch inflexible hamstrings, or simply to learn proper technique in their sport. If we can isolate and address the underlying issues behind this pain, we can prevent it from becoming a chronic and more serious problem for the child in the future.

Molly, 14

"I've been dancing since I was two years old, all kinds of dance: ballet, jazz, and tap. I'd had growing problems in the patellofemoral joint of my left knee for a while.

Then, in December, I was pushing myself and going to extra practices because I wanted to be in a higher group, and I heard this weird popping noise in my right knee. It hurt a lot right away, and kept swelling up. A piece of tissue, my plica, had gotten caught underneath my kneecap. I went to my doctor and he wanted to put me in surgery right away, but my mom thought he'd rushed into it and didn't want me to have it, so my friend Annamarie told me about the doctor she'd seen for her elbow and I went to him instead.

The new doctor said surgery was a last resort and put me in therapy. Icing helped with the swelling, but none of the anti-inflammatories worked, even the prescription ones. It hurt a lot, especially going up and down stairs at school. I did therapy for four and a half months, three times a week for an hour or an hour and a half. It was a lot of time, but it worked—I didn't have to get surgery and I'm back in dance.

Therapy was mostly about strengthening both knees. After I got the plica injury, I didn't do anything for almost a month, and when I finally got to the doctor, he told me that the muscles were so weak they could barely hold the kneecap in place. The left knee is still weaker than the right because it's been injured for so much longer, but they're both stronger than they used to be.

I also have really flat feet, which nobody had ever noticed before, so I went to a podiatrist to get fitted for orthotic inserts. I wear a brace on my right knee, the one with the plica, and that helped a lot. It's annoying, though—you wear a brace under your clothes and everybody asks you what's wrong with you.

I've cut down my dance class schedule because the doctor and my teachers wanted me to. I was doing six or seven classes a week before, and now I'm down to three. I'll probably only do four next year.

I'm not in therapy anymore, but I joined the gym where I did the therapy, and I do the home exercises. I'm glad I didn't have to have surgery—I would have been out longer, and I learned a lot in therapy about different ways to strengthen your knee and how to prevent further injury. It benefits you. I liked the people there, and I like the atmosphere at the gym. I'm going to continue doing the exercises and get my knees stronger so I can gradually increase the number of classes I'm taking."

Hip Problems

Children are subject to a range of hip problems that may present as knee problems. Some of these include Legge-Calve-Perthes disease, which is compromised blood supply to the head of the femur, sometimes known simply as Perthes disease; slipped capital femoral epiphysis (SCFE), where the top of the thighbone is in an abnormal position in the hip socket; as well as transient synovitis, inflammation of the tissues around the hip.

It's important that the physician check the patient for hip problems, even when the child is specifically complaining of knee pain. These problems can be easy to miss, and there are a number of anecdotal stories about unnecessary arthoscopic knee surgeries performed to address pain that was actually referred from the hip.

Growth Plate Injuries

Children's bones are still growing, which makes them particularly susceptible to injury to the growth plates. In a child, a strong ligament like the MCL attached to the growth plate area may withstand a traumatic force much better than the growth plate does, so many of the injuries that would show up as ligament injuries in an adult result as bone or growth plate injuries and fractures in children.

Osteochondritis Dissecans

Osteochondritis Dissecans occurs when a piece of the thighbone and its articular cartilage separate, either partially or completely, from the rest of the bone. The loose pieces of cartilage and bone can get trapped in the joint and cause locking and pain.

It may be linked to growth disturbances since it seems to happen most often among active adolescents and young adults. The knee is sore after activity, and may lock. RICE will help to reduce swelling, and the doctor may recommend a short period of crutches and immobilization and a longer period of modified activity for your child. Surgical options, such as debridement and cartilage grafting, may also be options.

Juvenile Arthritis

We tend to think of arthritis as a disease of the middle-aged and elderly, but this isn't always the case. The Arthritis Foundation estimates that 285,000 children have arthritis in the United States. Juvenile arthritis is inflammation of one or more joints in someone under fifteen years of age. Nobody knows what causes arthritis to strike a child; although there may be a genetic component involved, the condition does not appear to be hereditary.

As with adults, there are a wide variety of types. The most common is an autoimmune disease called juvenile rheumatoid arthritis, which can come on in different ways and it may have different symptoms. Many joints can be involved (usually large ones like the knee), and may be accompanied by fatigue, fever, skin rash, and other areas of inflammation.

Many of the treatment options available to adults with arthritis are also available for children, although drug dosages will be different and some drugs aren't approved for use in children. Surgery is rarely recommended until the child's growth has stopped. Physical therapy can help with pain, and may encourage more normal bone and joint growth as well.

There are physicians who specialize in pediatric rheumatology, and they can help parents and their arthritic children manage this disease. The American Juvenile Arthritis Organization (AJAO) is a council of the Arthritis Foundation devoted to serving the special needs of children, teens, and young adults with childhood rheumatic diseases and their families. They publish a wide range of literature on the topic, as well as sponsor conferences and summer camps for children with arthritis. You can find out about local chapters and get in touch with them through the Arthritis Foundation website, *www.arthritis.org*.

Meniscal Injury

In the adolescent, mensical injuries are most commonly associated with ligament injuries. Meniscal injuries in kids under fourteen are very unusual and usually linked to a congenital meniscal abnormality. An example is the *discoid meniscus*, which is usually thicker and a slightly different shape than a normal meniscus, and is most often seen on the lateral side (the outside of the leg). In most cases, this is totally asymptomatic, but some preadolescents and adolescents may begin to hear a snap in the knee when they walk, or have pain in the area of the meniscus laterally.

These knee injuries can be treated conservatively unless there is chronic pain or locking of the knee, in which case arthroscopic surgery may be used to neaten up the cartilage, normalize the shape of the meniscus, and treat any tear that is present.

A Note to Parents About Sports

Children's athletics have changed considerably. Instead of sandlot baseball and pickup basketball in someone's driveway, sports for kids have become considerably more formal and organized.

This increased level of sophistication is certainly making our children better athletes, and the improvement in equipment and training may even prevent injury. But this added formal dimension has a negative side. It takes sports and physical activity out of the everyday realm. A kid with energy to burn doesn't just run down the block to see who's free before dinner. You have to get a ride to a special facility that needs to be booked in advance, and there have to be a certain number of kids for an official game.

I applaud children's participation in organized sports, but I'm concerned that when physical activity becomes "a big deal," kids don't do as much of it, or learn to incorporate it into their lives. Without formal organization, they simply don't know what to do. This formalization has also led to increased competition, which is good in some ways, but can lead to coaches and parents living vicariously through young athletes, which can result in pushing them past what is safe and recommended.

I'd like to encourage parents to do what they can to bring physical activity back into children's lives in a more informal way, as well as supporting their more organized activities. Toss a ball with your kids in the yard, go bike riding or in-line skating with them in the park over the weekend, spend a hot Saturday playing at a friend's pool or at the beach. This will encourage your children to think of physical activity as something that's fun and integrated into their lives, not something that's restricted to uniformed competition in a sports facility.

Our children's future well-being is determined, in large part, by their level of physical activity when they're young. Learning good exercise habits and becoming accustomed to a comfortable level of physical activity at an early age will have a positive impact on the rest of their lives. An active child is much more likely to become an active adult— and is less likely to be overweight or obese, and to develop diabetes and cardiovascular disease. Don't allow this important effort to be derailed by knee pain: address your child's complaints early and the underlying issues causing them.

CHAPTER SEVENTEEN

SPECIAL CONCERNS

The Elderly

Fifteen years ago, the most common musculoskeletal complaint among the elderly was unquestionably arthritis, but this has changed dramatically over the last decade. Older people are staying active longer, and that means better health in general. It also means that I'm seeing more sports- and activity-related injuries in the older population. It's not just happening in my practice: a U.S. Consumer Product Safety Commission (CPSC) report released in 1998 showed that from 1990 to 1996, sports-related injuries to persons 65 and older increased 54 percent. Sports-related injuries to persons 75 and older increased by 29 percent.

This is only becoming a bigger issue as the baby boomers get older. Another CPSC report, this one from April 2000, showed that there was a 33 percent increase from 1991 to 1998 in sports-related injuries among people ages 35 to 54. This population is getting *more*, not less active as they head into their retirement years.

Exercise works to combat a number of the issues that arise as we age: it helps to keep stiff joints mobile, tight muscles flexible, and brittle bones strong. Many of the maladies we used to think were an inevitable result of aging are the result of the sedentary behavior that used to be forced on the elderly.

But given these growing sports-injury numbers among the elderly, it's clear that we're going to have to change the way we think about geriatric sports medicine to make sure that we're giving people the best treatment possible. The elderly have a host of special concerns, and neglecting these issues means that they're often misdiagnosed and mistreated. And because older people are slower to heal, they can be more difficult to rehabilitate.

Keeping Safe

The best medicine is prevention, and there is much that older people can do to take precautions and keep their knees safe.

See your doctor. The American College of Sports Medicine recommends that anyone over forty see their doctor for evaluation before beginning a new exercise program. You want to make sure that your cardiovascular system is in adequate shape to handle the stress of a workout. Your doctor can also give you advice, specific to your case, on ways to protect previous injury sites or to accommodate any medical issues you might have.

Warm up and cool down. Older athletes do have stiffer muscles and joints, and can benefit from a longer transition period in and out of exercise. Warm up for ten or fifteen minutes, stretch well, and then do your activity. Give yourself a little longer to cool down as well.

Stay trim. It's easier to gain weight as we get older, and harder to take it off once it's on. But carrying extra weight is hard on the joints, so it becomes even more important to watch our waistlines as we age.

Be strong. Our muscles naturally weaken as the body gets older, so you may have to work harder and with more focus on strengthening parts of the body that used to stay strong without effort.

Stay hydrated. Older people dehydrate faster than younger people do, and they're more susceptible to altitude sickness and heat exhaustion, so make sure you're consuming enough water, especially when you're exercising.

Treating the Elderly

As you've seen over the course of this book, age is necessarily a factor that we take into consideration when we're discussing treatment options.

We've talked about the importance of treating the whole patient, and this is especially true in the case of the elderly. For instance, an elderly person is more likely to have overlapping medical issues—other injuries and other medications to take into account. When we're treating an elderly person, even someone who's extremely independent, we need to think more about issues of daily living: transportation, the home or assisted living environment.

Arthritis

Arthritis is one of the most significant problems in an elderly population, and it's something that I've talked about at great length in this book. One of the things to be aware of is that knee pain in the elderly may actually be pain referred from an arthritic hip, so that's something that your doctor should check thoroughly before treating your knee pain.

A controversial study done at the Houston Veteran's Administration Medical Center and published in the prestigious *New England Journal of Medicine* showed that arthroscopic debridement surgeries, which are performed on hundreds of thousands of senior citizens a year in order to alleviate pain from osteoarthritis, didn't help any more than a placebo surgery did.

You have to be careful when you're reading these studies; they can be interpreted in a multitude of ways. Arthroscopy is certainly not "the answer" to arthritis, but it may address related meniscus issues, especially if the knee is locking—and that can be valuable. No, it's probably not worth the risks of surgery to get the month or two of pain relief that you'll get from simply washing out the joint, but if there are loose bodies causing pain and causing the knee to give way, then it may be a very good idea to address these issues surgically. This is why it's so important to decide each case on a patient-by-patient basis.

The Elderly in Rehab

Older people take longer to get better—it's just true. As we age, our bodies are not only less resilient and therefore more prone to injury but they're slower to heal.

There's a silver lining to this cloud, which is that elderly people often have more time. You may be retired, or working on a reduced schedule, and that means you have extra time and energy to give to your rehab. Make it part of your routine, give it the time you need, and you'll find yourself making up whatever you've lost in natural muscle strength and flexibility.

Make sure that your physical therapist has experience in rehabilitating elderly people, and if your intention is to return to sports, make sure that's clear at the very beginning of the relationship.

CHAPTER EIGHTEEN

SPECIAL CONCERNS

The Disabled

Although there is an enormous disabled population in the United States, this community is rarely addressed directly in relation to knee pain and injury.

Since there are so many types of disability, it's difficult to adequately and accurately discuss the group as a whole in specific terms. But there are some issues that I'd like to highlight. Let's take a step back: how do we define disability?

The Americans with Disabilities Act (ADA) and Section 504 of the Rehabilitation Act of 1973, defines disability as:

A physical or mental impairment that substantially limits one or more of the major life activities typically performed by an individual such as caring for one's self, performing manual tasks, walking, seeing, hearing, and working.

Obviously, this is vague. First of all, what is a "physical impairment"? It's a disorder that affects one or more of the following systems: neurological, musculoskeletal, respiratory, cardiovascular, endocrine, reproductive, digestive, genitourinary, blood and lymph systems, the sense organs, or the skin. And "substantially limits"—what does that mean? It means that you're unable to perform, or substantially limited compared to an average person.

Since knee pain and injury can further exacerbate a disability, or actually cause one even if only temporarily, it's essential for us to address this issue.

Knee pain is a considerable problem for someone who's already functioning with only one leg, for example. If something goes wrong on their "good side," then their ability to function is severely compromised. Many above-the-knee amputee cyclists don't use a prosthetic, so if something is off with the leg they use to cycle with, they can't participate in their sport. Below-the-knee amputees face other risks: hyperextension knee injuries can result from the body's forward momentum while it's moving over the fixed prosthesis. Impact injuries also frequently occur to amputees.

Paraplegics have an additional set of problems. If you use your lower body to balance as you transfer from a chair to a bed to a wheelchair, then a knee problem can affect your stability during the transfer and lead to more serious injury. Also, the loss of muscle tone that may accompany a lower-extremity disability may increase your risk of injury; by the same token, the increase in muscle tone as a result of spasm can also decrease stability and increase the likelihood of injury.

So how can we prevent a knee crisis in the disabled community?

Using the proper equipment and ensuring that it's in good working order is a first priority for everyone who participates in a sport or activity. Have your wheelchair checked often for wear. And wear knee pads, especially when playing sports like basketball where there's a fairly high risk that you'll be thrown from your chair.

Tanya, 36

"I'm a below-the-knee amputee on the left side, and I've been running consistently and competitively since 1987.

There are a million issues confronting a high-level amputee athlete, but one of the biggest ones is prosthetics. You really depend on your equipment, much more than most athletes. And it's a hard road: although they're miles ahead of where they were, these devices simply aren't as good as they might be. It's always going to be a little bit of an imprecise science, requiring a lot of attention from the athlete: the parts wear out, they don't fit well, your needs change, etc.

The right prosthetic makes an enormous difference—it can turn a 10-minute mile into a 7:30 mile without any appreciable change in effort. If you're competing in something like the Paralympics, which is extremely competitive, hundredths of a second make a difference. And it's hard for a disabled athlete to get that perfect feeling, the perfect fit every time; it's hard to get redundancy. You're always working out systems, and whenever something gets changed, you have to start back at square one.

A good relationship with a really talented prosthetist is essential. I finally found someone I feel comfortable with, someone who will listen to what I want and work with me. It requires creativity on their part. For instance, it turns out that the best foot for me is actually one designed for an active 200-pound man, not the one designed for an active 115-pound woman.

A number of my injuries have had to do with my prosthetic and the way I was using it. Runners should change their shoes every 250 miles. The problem is that nobody knows how often you should change your foot. My background is in physics and engineering, so I keep good logs and give my prosthetist good feedback. The more high-end athletes that do this, the better the devices are going to get. But there are a lot of variables, and sometimes you don't know until you're injured. My most recent injury was a bout with iliotibial band syndrome, and I think it had a lot to do with wearing out my foot. I was racing a lot last year, and the foot lost stiffness, and my hip was dipping. My first serious injury, a foot injury, was undoubtedly the result of a poor foot fit. And I kept running through the pain, which is something I won't do again.

The other thing to remember is that what's comfortable isn't always what's best for you. I like to run on a softer foot, but it's not as good for me. My prosthetist can adjust the alignment of my foot, and when he does, I'm suddenly working completely different muscles. I know that I have a bad habit of inwardly rotating my prosthetic side from the hip. If the foot is aligned one way, it's easier for me to run, but that weak area in my hip isn't working. If the foot is aligned another way, it forces me to use the muscles that are weak, but it makes me work harder. And as I get fitter, the alignment needs to continue to change, which adds another complication to going in and out of a running season.

The big problem with prosthetics is that they're really, really expensive: money is definitely the limiting factor. It means that sometimes you know your foot is going south, and you can't get the workout you want unless you can afford another one—or risk injury. And it takes forever. The new foot I just got took a month to make, because they can only make one of them at a time.

I know a lot of disabled athletes who stop working out because they can't deal with keeping up with the prosthetic end of it. I was doing a lot of cycling as part of my cross-training a few years back, and I cut back on my training because my calf muscles were getting really big and it was interfering with the fit of my prosthetic.

I love running, and my goal is to run for the rest of my life. I'm also a mountain climber, and I want to do that for the rest of my life too. My ultimate goal has to be to stay healthy so I can keep doing those things. Sometimes that may mean that I don't get the workout I want because something feels off—the fit isn't working the way it should, or I'm huffing and puffing because the foot isn't pushing back. As aggravating as that inconsistency is, you have to learn when to back off and when to push."

Everyone should also pay attention to their bodies and report changes to their doctors. Even people with neurological deficits—people who can't feel their lower bodies, for instance—get clues that there's a problem if they pay close attention. Those clues may not be pain, but the body somehow knows that something's not right. You may be experiencing more spasms than usual on one side, for instance, and if you communicate that to your doctor, then he can play detective and go looking for the cause. It might be a hairline fracture, for instance, or a meniscal tear.

It's imperative that you maintain as much muscle function as possible, because that will enable you to function to your maximum degree. It might mean extra work to make small gains, but it's important to set goals and meet them, and to team up with a good physical therapist who will help you meet those goals. Don't forget to work daily on increasing your flexibility as well.

As with everyone, exercise and activity are among the best ways to prevent and recover from knee injury—regular exercise is good for the body and good for the mind. If you're interested in getting involved, I'd encourage you to get in touch with World TEAM (The Exceptional Athlete Matters) Sports, *www.worldteamsports.org*, a nonprofit organization that integrates disability and ability through inclusion, teamwork, and sports. I have been involved in this organization since 1993. They hold multiple events in the United States and abroad to bring disabled and abled athletes and non-athletes together in activities of sport to recognize the importance of one human being helping another.

Every disability is different, and the way that you adapt and react to your disability is different. It's imperative to have a good working relationship with your doctor. Certainly, disabled does not mean unable. To quote a disabled adolescent from Russia's heartland, who spoke no English: "We all have the human spirit, abled and disabled. It's just the containers of our spirit that are different."

PART VI

CONCLUSION

THE FUTURE
LOOKS BRIGHT

Our best defense against the crisis of knee pain and injury is a good offense. Whether you've experienced knee pain and injury yourself, or you're looking to help someone else—a child, a spouse, a parent—you've taken an important first step to combat the knee crisis in your life simply by reading this book.

It's essential that we continue to educate ourselves about the problems that confront our knees and the range of possible solutions to those problems. A sports medicine icon and my mentor, Dr. Jack Hughston, is known for saying, "When you're green, you're still growing; when you're ripe, you're next to rotten." In other words, we have to keep learning and evolving to stay alive—when we think we know everything there is to know, we stagnate.

This goes for both physicians and their patients. There have been spectacular developments in the sports medicine field, and there is much to be excited about on the horizon. Imaging technology is improving by leaps and bounds, which will make it easier for your doctor to tell, with a tremendous degree of accuracy, what's wrong with you. Surgical techniques, particularly in the areas of bone, cartilage, muscle, and tendon biology, are developing rapidly and hold tremendous promise for knee pain sufferers. Rehabilitation strategies, designed to get you back to a high level of activity as swiftly and painlessly as possible, continue to gain in sophistication. New technologies and solutions emerge daily.

Patients are also becoming better educated about their knees and more involved in their treatment, to great effect. The better educated you are, the better you'll be able to manage your risk, participate in treatment decisions, and the more realistic your expectations will be for your recovery. The Internet and books like this one offer a wealth of information and community resources to people with knee pain. Many patients have sought out alternative therapies, and as a result, these therapies are becoming more and more integrated into conventional medicine.

As exciting as these developments are, it's also important to keep the fundamentals in sight. There's no technology that can replace open, honest, patient-doctor communication, and the information that a doctor can gather from a detailed medical history and hands-on manipulation of the leg. And there's no information that you can find on the Internet that can replace being taken care of by someone with whom you have a relationship. These are integral parts of the healing equation, and I hope that over the course of this book you've developed some skills to address your own knee crisis proactively.

Finally, I find myself returning to this concept of balance, and if there's one central concept that I'd like you to take from this book, it's this: when we allow ourselves to fall out of balance, we get into trouble. Balance—between work and play; between rest and activity; between the muscle groups at the front and the back of the body, and the muscle groups on the inside and the outside of the leg; between self-education and developing and maintaining a relationship with a trusted professional—all of these things play a role in our ability to prevent injury and to heal and recover efficiently.

Every knee injury may be a crisis, but it doesn't have to be a permanently debilitating one. The more you know, the more empowered you'll be to participate in your care, so educate yourself, request a high level of care, and commit yourself to rehabilitation, and you'll be rewarded by your results.

Appendix

Personal Patient Information

Treatment for a knee injury can take place over a long period of time. Here we've provided you with a place to keep all of your own personal patient records, so that all the information is easily accessible in one place and you can refer back to it if you need it.

My Information

Date of Birth: _____

Sex: _____

Health history: _____

_____

_____

_____

My Doctor

Name: _____

Address: _____

_____

Phone Number: _____

My Injury

Date: _____

History of Injury:_____

_____

_____

_____

_____

Diagnostic Tests Performed (MRI, X ray, etc.): _____

_____

_____

_____

_____

_____

_____

_____

Diagnosis:_____

_____

_____

_____

_____

_____

Treatment Options: _____

_____

_____

_____

_____

Questions & Answers:_____

_____

_____

_____

_____

_____

Chosen Treatment:_____

_____

_____

_____

_____

Comfort Measures: _____

_____

_____

_____

Medications (recommended or prescribed):_____

_____

_____

Doctor's Visit Log

Date: _____

Reason for Visit:_____

Conclusion: _____

_____

_____

Braces, Prosthetics, Other Products Used: _____

_____

_____

My Surgery

Date: _____

Surgeon: _____

Hospital:_____

Procedure performed: _____

_____

Additional Notes/Comments: _____

_____

My Physical Therapy

Note: You may want to photocopy the following pages before writing on them to ensure that you don't run out of room.

Physical Therapist: _____

Telephone Number: _____

Address of Facility: _____

_____

Physical Therapy Sessions: _____

Homework Assignments: _____

_____

_____

DATE	EXERCISE	NUMBER OF REPS	NUMBER OF SETS

DATE	EXERCISE	NUMBER OF REPS	NUMBER OF SETS

My Personal Knee Health Program

Exercises, diet, alternative treatments;
what worked for me, and what didn't:_____

_____

_____

_____

_____

_____

_____

My Personal Knee Health Progress Report

My personal milestones and setbacks: _____

_____

_____

_____

_____

_____

_____

_____

GLOSSARY

ACL: anterior cruciate ligament, one of the ligaments that run through the center of the knee joint.

Alignment: the way the elements of the legs line up in relation to one another.

Allograft: a graft taken from tissue that comes from someone or somewhere else.

Arthritis: inflammation of the joint.

Arthroscopy: surgical technique in which a tiny camera is inserted into the leg so that the surgeon can see the inside of the knee without making a major incision.

Articular cartilage: rubbery, protective cartilage coating the end of bones.

Aspiration: inserting a needle into the joint in order to remove some of the fluid inside, used both a diagnosis and a treatment.

Autograft: a graft made of tissue taken from inside the patient.

Bursa: small, protective, fluid-filled sacs found all over the body, often where the tendons connect to the bones.

Capsaicin: the compound that makes chili peppers spicy.

Cartilage: rubbery form of tissue that protects the bones in the knee.

Condyle: round knob at the end of the femur.

Crepitus: crunching sound or feeling accompanying movement of the knee.

Debridement: an arthroscopic procedure to remove damaged cartilage and bone from the knee.

Female athlete triad: the combination of an eating disorder such as bulimia or anorexia combined with an infrequent or absent menstrual cycle, and bone loss.

Femur: the thighbone.

Fibula: bone on the outside of the lower leg.

Genu valgus: knock-kneed.

Genu varus: bowlegged.

Hamstring: three major muscles at the back of the thigh.

Hemoarthrosis: bleeding into the joint.

Hyperlaxity: loose-jointedness.

Iliotibial band: the combined muscle-tendon package that stretches all the way from the ilium (pelvis) to the tibia (shinbone).

Intercondylar notch: the space between the round knobs at the end of the femur.

Kinesthetic awareness: the ability to accurately perceive a limb's movement in space.

Lateral release: an arthroscopic procedure in which the lateral retinaculum is cut and released.

Lateral retinaculum: system of supporting soft tissue on the outside of the patella.

Ligament: the tissue connecting bone to bone.

McConnell taping: a method of taping the patella in place.

Meniscus: rounded, rubbery cartilage cushions between the thighbone and the shinbone.

Miserable malalignment syndrome: a combination of femoral anteversion, knock knees, externally rotated tibias, and flatfeet.

MRI: a diagnostic test that uses magnetic and radio waves to produce images of tissues inside the body.

NSAIDs: Non-steroidal anti-inflammatory drugs, available both over-the-counter and by prescription, that relieve pain and fight inflammation.

Orthotics: any appliance attached to a limb that improves the function of that limb; often a shoe insert or a brace to correct alignment.

Osteochondral fracture: displacement of the bone and sometimes the cartilage.

Patella: kneecap.

Plica: fold in the synovial lining.

Plyometrics: high-velocity drills designed to increase speed and strength.

Pronate: the inward turning of the ankle and foot, often associated with flatfeet.

Proprioception: understanding of where your limbs are in space.

Relative rest: taking the load off the joint without immobilizing it by modifying activity.

RICE: R(est), I(ce), C (ompression), and E(levation).

Q angle: the measure of the alignment between the pelvis, leg, and foot.

Quadriceps: the large muscle group on the top of the thigh.

Subluxation: a partial dislocation of the kneecap.

Supinate: the tendency of the ankle and foot to roll outward, often associated with high arches.

Synovium: the lining of the balloon-like capsule that surrounds the knee.

Tendon: the tissue connecting muscle to bone.

Tibia: shinbone.

Tibial tuberosity: the bony protrusion below the center of the kneecap.

Theater knee: a knee that is stiff after inactivity or sitting for a long time.

Trochlear groove: the groove in the thighbone that allows the patella to move.

Valgus: turned outward.

Varus: turned inward.

VMO: vastus medialis, the inner quadriceps muscle.

X ray: a diagnostic test that uses electromagnetic beams to produce images of tissues inside the body.

INDEX